Working on Wicked Problems

Komla Tsey

Working on Wicked Problems

A Strengths-based Approach to
Research Engagement and Impact

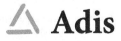

Komla Tsey
James Cook University
Cairns
QLD
Australia

ISBN 978-3-030-22323-6   ISBN 978-3-030-22325-0   (eBook)
https://doi.org/10.1007/978-3-030-22325-0

This Adis imprint is published by the registered company Springer Nature Switzerland AG
The registered company address is: Gewerbestrasse 11, 6330 Cham, Switzerland

Foreword

'Emotional' and 'moving' are not words one may usually associate with the process of research. In my academic career, however, I have experienced many extremes and seen the power and impact that research (and individual researchers) can have when they engage genuinely and honestly with their research communities. One of the most inspiring and moving moments of my research career took place in the small Aboriginal community of Yarrabah, a seaside town just south of Cairns in Far Northern Australia, at the culmination of a research project on which Professor Komla Tsey and I were co-leaders. Professor Tsey and I were in Yarrabah for the opening of an international mental health conference in 2006. The community was to showcase its successful suicide prevention activities, particularly the roles and contributions of Family Wellbeing and Men's Group research. The local men's dance group, Yabba Bimbie, performed a moving 'research dance' on the opening day of the conference, which involved research collaborators from James Cook University (JCU), the University of Queensland (UQ) and the Gurriny Yealamucka Health Service Aboriginal Corporation (GYHSAC). The dance referenced a traditional healing pool called 'Yealamucka' and represented the healing process within social health programmes. The dance also expressed the relationship between the community and universities.

A lead dancer enacted the experience of being down and out on the streets—plagued by drugs, alcohol and mental health problems—crying out for help and healing for his body, soul and spirit. The JCU-UQ team and GYHSAC staff members stood within the circle of dancers and reached out their hands and arms to assist this man in need. Their support enabled him to lift himself out of despair. As the lead dancer moved towards them, the supporters stepped aside to give him space. The other dancers followed. They were all passing through Yealamucka. Together, they reached a place where they were able to work as a group to take greater control and responsibility and to realise the vision they had for themselves as men, for their families and for the Yarrabah community. No longer did they need alcohol or drugs to live life. In making this change, they became role models.

The lead dancer explained that the name of the health service, Gurriny Yealamucka, had important historical significance. Traditionally, people had gone to the healing waters, Yealamucka, if they were sick or wanted to maintain good health. At this healing pool, people would sing and dance and then bathe in the water to be healed by the spirit of the land. The involvement of Gurriny Yealamucka staff symbolised the responsibility the new health service had assumed for community healing through the Men's Group, Women's Group and youth programmes. The JCU and UQ researchers had facilitated and supported this transition. The performance reflected a transformation in the emphasis and methodology of applied research within Indigenous communities. This combination of the traditional way and the European way was the essence of reconciliation.

The Yarrabah research collaboration, which the research dance movingly depicted, formed part of a 10-year programme of empowerment research (2001–2010) which started at UQ and later transferred with the staff to JCU. As I was a co-leader of the research programme, the research dance was, for me, the most powerful portrayal of a true partnership between community and researchers. It was both an emotional and a spiritual experience to see a group of Aboriginal men celebrating and honouring the contribution of research, not only to suicide prevention within their community but also to the role research collaboration was playing in realising the community's vision of building their own comprehensive community-controlled primary health-care service. The performance inspired me; Komla Tsey, co-leader of the research programme; and Leslie Baird, the manager of the fledgling community-controlled health service, to write about our experiences in engaging in research with communities. Leslie has presented widely on his experiences, and I am delighted that Komla has finally written this long-awaited book on his experience of working not only with Aboriginal communities but also with his own community in Africa.

This book is relevant for anyone involved in the complex world of research, particularly social research. For researchers, it gives them practical ideas about how to engage communities, especially when dealing with emotionally sensitive topics such as suicide prevention. For community leaders and managers of organisations, it helps them to consider proactive steps they can take to make research serve their needs and aspirations. For funding bodies, including philanthropic organisations, it helps them to learn about the need to trust communities and support promising interventions over longer 10- to 20-year periods in order to translate the rhetoric of empowerment into reality.

Yvonne Cadet-James
James Cook University
Douglas, QLD, Australia

Apunipima Cape York Health Council
Bungalow, QLD, Australia

Bibliography

Cadet-James, Y., James, R. A., McGinty, S., & McGregor, R. (2017). *Gugu Badhun: People of the Valley of Lagoons*. Canberra: Aboriginal Studies Press.

Mayo, K., & Tsey, K. (2009). Research dancing: reflections on the relationships between university-based researchers and community-based researchers at Gurriny Yealamucka Health Services Aboriginal Corporation, Yarrabah. Darwin: Cooperative Research Centre for Aboriginal Health.

Mayo, K., Tsey, K., & Empowerment Research Team. (2009). The research dance: University and community research collaborations at Yarrabah, North Queensland, Australia. *Health & Social Care in the Community, 17*(2), 133–140.

Preface

The impetus for this book stems from a growing expectation worldwide that researchers must be able to demonstrate, qualify and quantify the impact of their research on society. It is quite an endeavour to demonstrate the impact of a particular project on a society. I have given much thought to the idea of impact and completed significant work in demonstrating the impact of my own work. For me, as a social researcher, my questions and my answers about impact have consistently returned to one significant aspect of social research projects—research engagement. Researchers, particularly those based in universities, are engaging with industry and community partners more often in order to demonstrate the societal impact of their work. Working across different societal sectors, like human services or remote communities, requires a distinctive skillset that is vastly different from the stereotype of a researcher from days gone by: the obsessive scholar working in solitude. Research engagement, especially cross-sector research engagement, has not, in itself, been subject to extensive scholarly investigation. It is difficult to find in-depth cases, stories or research papers that describe how individual researchers engage with their research communities. The challenges and opportunities associated with research engagement have not been addressed in detail either. To date, the scholarly literature about research engagement and impact has focused on the development of research impact tools, types of research impact and development of impact case studies and measurable indicators of engagement, such as the number of industry grants received by university researchers. These facts and figures, although important, tell us little about the *how* of research engagement and about the dynamics and messiness of the engagement process. They neither are helpful in understanding how engagement may result in impact for society nor do they shed light on the competencies required for effective engagement and impact assessment.

My aim in writing this book is to share aspects of my journey as a researcher, from the small village in Ghana where I first began asking big questions to my current career as a university researcher in Australia. I focus on *wicked problems* as the lens through which to share my research experience to convey the message that there are no magic bullets for solving the most complex and difficult social problems. The best we can do as researchers is to contribute to a better understanding of problems and ways to approach them, knowing very well that our efforts may only help to achieve limited answers or partial solutions. The focus on wicked problems is also to highlight the importance of the so-called twenty-first-century or global soft skills and the simple and effective ways I have used to foster the development of these capabilities in many people of different ages, genders and cultural backgrounds.

I have chosen a case study approach. In each chapter, I have chosen and told a story from my research experience to illustrate a particular enabling factor or an attribute of research engagement and impact. *Case study* is an approach to research that investigates a phenomenon within its real-life situation. Case studies are valuable in monitoring and assessing research engagement and impact because they provide a wide and rounded perspective that can address attribution and the relative contribution of the research to the observed impact. Case studies usually use both quantitative and qualitative approaches. They tend to appraise a broader concept of impact than numbers alone; with case studies, you may investigate various dimensions of the economic, social and environmental returns from research, thereby capturing more intangible benefits such as research partner experience, satisfaction and wellbeing.

A significant part of my research career to date has taken place in and for Aboriginal and Torres Strait Islander communities. I have learnt much about engagement and collaborative ways of working from people and colleagues in these communities. I respectfully use the term 'Aboriginal' when discussing events that took place in Central Australia or Yarrabah, but when talking about Australia as a whole, where I also worked with Torres Strait Islander people, I use the term 'Indigenous'. My research career has taken me to urban, rural, remote and interesting parts of Australia, Africa and beyond, where I have worked on messy and complicated problems related to death, love, sex and alcohol abuse among other things. I have pondered the sustainable disposal of dead bodies of loved ones in Ghana. I have assisted a remote Aboriginal community to research and tackle the striptease-sex tourism in their town. I have listened to stories of family breakdown and recovery and strength. I have observed the resilience, creativity and determination with which a rural Aboriginal community, Yarrabah in north Queensland, implemented a range of long-term whole-of-community crisis and preventative interventions to reduce suicide rates among young people. As I have engaged communities of people in research for more than 30 years, I have experienced many wonderful moments as well as false starts and falls. I want to share the stories and knowledge I have gained from my experiences. Through this reflection, I hope to highlight some of the attributes, competencies and approaches needed by research students and community researchers to gain confidence and become more effective.

Cairns, QLD, Australia   Komla Tsey

Acknowledgements

This book took no more than 6 months to write, but the underpinning projects and activities occurred over a period of 40 years in a wide variety of settings across Ghana, Australia, Papua New Guinea, China and Timor-Leste. As I wrote each chapter, the many ways in which individuals, organisations and, in some cases, whole communities have supported my work over the years became obvious to me. Some people gave me professional opportunities, some collaborated with me, some assisted me, and some gave me friendship and affection, while others challenged me to do better. My very special thanks go to the following: Afua Tsey, Felix Kortortsie, FMK Asamoah, Yao Anka, Charlie Akotiakuma, Koku W Adufutse, Yaya Owusu, Abra Gavua, Yao Addo-Fenning, Evelyn Mawuli Atsodibuor, Victor Komla Abotsi, Victor Mensah, Inez Sutton, FK Ameka, Stephanie Short, Annekathrin Schmid, John Boffa, Chris George, Jayne Schoefield, Pat Anderson, William Tilmouth, John Mathews, Mick Gooda, Romlie Mokak, Lyn Brodie, Anne Every, Elaine Williams, Emma Hopkins, Ernest Hunter, Ross Sparks, Robyn McDermott, Leslie Baird, Bradley Baird, David Paterson, Ruth Fagan, Karen Dini-Paul, Cleaveland Fagan, Mary Whiteside, Yvonne Cadet-James, Theresa Gibson, Audrey Deemal, Rachael Ham, Elizabeth Pearson, Mark Wenitong, Janya McCalman, Roxanne Bainbridge, Andrew Wilson, Anthony Shakeshaft, Melissa Haswell, Radhika Santhanam, Chris Doran, Ross Bailie, Cath Brown, Marion Heyeres, Irina Kinchin, Helen Klieve, Felecia Watkin, Lynda Ah Mat, Patricia Dudgeon, Alwin Chong, Rick Spear, Ines Zuchowski, Robyn Moylan, Kieran Smith, Zona Gabriel, Nigel Millgate, Ben Cheniart, Russel Kitau, Li Yan, Yang Yinghong, Carrie Lui, Hua Jiang, Jenny Liangjun Zuo, John Grundy, Katrina Keith, Leigh-Ann Onnis, Taha Hunter, Niru Perera, Astri Baker, Sarah Gosling, Kirsty Smith, Deborah Fisher, Suzanne Gibson, Priscilla Akpene Addo, Akpene Attakey and Kat Cacavas. I thank the Aboriginal Employment Development Branch for their insight in creating the Family Wellbeing programme and all the Family Wellbeing participants for sharing their stories with me over the years. I also thank the NHMRC-funded Centre for Research Excellence in Integrated Quality Improvement for their in-kind support. Annie, my partner, I thank you for your love, for your intellectual curiosity and for putting up with my weird working hours. Kwame, Sena, Kafui, Amenyo and Novi, thank you for your love and for making fun of my working habits. Anne Constantine, Gloria Webb and Marnie Hitchins, thank you so much for your wonderful editing skills. As the Botoku people say, 'akpe gaa de nami loo', a big thank you to you all!

About This Book

This book is for researchers and students looking for ways to engage communities and industry in research. It is also written for community leaders, philanthropists and managers of organisations interested in building mutually beneficial partnerships with researchers, or training their own researchers. To this end, I hope that the readers of this book will appreciate that in their own way, whether big or small, they will be able to make research more meaningful by genuinely and honestly engaging with the communities of people with whom they work with. I hope that an auto-ethnography or personal narrative approach will throw light on the factors that lead to positive research engagement and help researchers to avoid some of my pitfalls.

Each chapter is presented as a stand-alone story about a particular factor contributing to research engagement and can be read as such. In choosing my stories, I reviewed dozens of projects in which I had been involved over the years. I chose to include a story as a case study if it highlighted a particular enabling factor, and I gave preference to projects where the publication on which the story was based was freely available in the public domain so that the interested readers could find more context and background to the work. Several case studies from one project were selected because I see a strong need for researchers to work with the same communities over time in order to truly demonstrate the impact of their research. Each chapter represents one part of the complex jigsaw puzzle that is research engagement. Read together, these small case studies tell a bigger story about a researcher trying to make a difference—to have an impact. In this way, I propose a strengths-based facilitation framework to inform more effective research engagement and impact.

Contents

About the Author

Komla Tsey lives in the Far North of Australia. His work centres on the identification and analysis of government policy, local community action and social and cultural norms that enable individuals, families and communities to achieve better health. He is a tropical leader in Education for Social Sustainability at James Cook University's The Cairns Institute. He has a broad research interest in the social determinants of health or the analysis of why some groups of people are healthy and others are not.

Komla was born and educated in Ghana. After earning a Bachelor of Arts (Honours) from the University of Ghana in 1980, he studied a Doctor of Philosophy in Social Science (Economic History) at Glasgow University, Scotland; his thesis examined the social, economic and health consequences of British colonial railway investments in Ghana. He returned to the University of Ghana after completing his PhD, lecturing and developing partnerships with rural communities as a participant observer/researcher in long-term development projects aimed at improving access to facilities such as schools, health services, electricity, water and sanitation.

Since the 1990s, Komla has been living in Australia, researching health and well-being, primarily with Aboriginal organisations and communities. He continues to undertake longitudinal studies of rural development in Ghana. His research and development activities have also taken him to Papua New Guinea, China and Timor-Leste. As part of his commitment to research translation, he teaches the following short courses for researchers, programme managers, front-line workers and community groups: Introduction to Research Engagement and Impact, Building 'Soft Skills' for Community Engagement and Introduction to the Family Wellbeing Empowerment program. With all of his courses, he provides follow-up support tailored to the needs of participants.

Contact: komla.tsey@jcu.edu.au for further information.

Aiming for Relevance: Early Experiences of Community Engagement in Ghana

Abstract

Education and research, no matter how interesting, are of limited value unless they are relevant to the needs and aspirations of people. A useful starting point for a researcher seeking to make their work relevant to their community is to pose a series of questions: Who is my research community? What are their needs and aspirations? How can my research support those needs and aspirations? In this first chapter, I describe the start of my research journey and my realisation that relevance is the key to research. I use anecdotes from my school days in Ghana, West Africa, to show how my early search for meaning, purpose and relevance in my home village set me on a path to becoming a university researcher.

When I think about engaging communities of people in research, anecdotes from my school days come to mind. I was born and completed primary school in the village of Botoku, in south-east Ghana. Like many rural and remote communities all over the world, there was no high school in my Ghanaian village. The only way to go to high school was to go away to boarding school or stay with family or friends in town. So, at the age of about 13, I left the village to further my education. It was clear in my mind, even before I went to high school, that I was going to be a lawyer. I was aware that law was expensive to study. So my plan was to complete high school on scholarship, go to university for a bachelor's degree and then secure a job as high school teacher in the city and study law part-time. I had it all mapped out!

In my holidays, like many of my classmates, I returned to the village and worked in the field with my parents. I recall my father asking me what we were learning at school. Perhaps I thought that, since my parents had not been to school, they would not understand, I found myself struggling to find anything to say that I thought would make sense to them. My father was a small-built man and a persistent, determined questioner who did not shy away from speaking his mind. He was not prepared to take silence for an answer. When I failed to answer his question for a third time, he gently but firmly said to me: 'Look, our son, if we send you to boarding school, and you cannot come back and make what you are learning relevant to the needs and aspirations of people in this village, then what is the point of sending you to school? You may as well come back to join us here and till the soil'. As someone who did not particularly like working in the field, I saw education as my escape from subsistence farming. The idea of rejoining my family in the village to 'till the soil' horrified me, and I began to ask myself exactly how I could make my learning relevant.

One of my earliest attempts to make what I was learning relevant was to become a letter writer in my village. At that time in Botoku, most adults had grown up under British colonial rule and very few people could read or write. I wrote official letters on behalf of the chiefs and elders to government departments and politicians to lobby for education, health and other community development resources. I wrote letters regarding compensation claims to lawyers on behalf of families in Botoku whose lands had been inundated by the construction of a major hydroelectric dam. But the letters that made the most lasting impression on me were the private ones, dictated mainly by women who wanted to send word from home to husbands or fiancés who had gone to distant urban centres in search of employment and education opportunities. This was long before the advent of mobile phones. As the letter writer, I was the primary conduit of communication between people moving away from the village and the families they left behind. Every now and then, a letter would arrive, delivered by a Botoku person visiting home or, less frequently, via the post. A typical letter from the men would start by asking how everybody was. They would say whether they had found a job, provide an update on efforts to secure a deposit to rent a room and end by saying when they may expect to send for the family to come and join them. I would read the letter to the woman who, in turn, would dictate her reply to me. Again, the letter would be very informational and straightforward. The woman would state how everybody was doing at home, whether any of the children had been sick, and offer thanks for any money sent with the letter.

As a child, I had loved the Ananse folklore stories told in my village. *Ananse* means spider, a creature that in Ghanaian mythology is reputed to be clever. Ananse stories were full of intrigue, love, passion, determination and loyalty. In contrast, I found the letters I was reading aloud and writing in return so very functional, unsentimental and totally lacking in passion, warmth or affection. Based upon my love of Ananse stories, I began spicing up the letters the women were dictating to me, a little bit at a time. I might end the letters with *mele susuo kakaka*, meaning 'I am missing you very much!' or *melo wo kakaka*, meaning 'I love you very much'. As a matter of course, I read every letter back to the women to ensure I conveyed the right messages. When I got to the end of a letter, where I had embellished a little, the women would say, 'You cheeky boy, Komla. Did I ask you to write that?' I would say, 'Sorry, I'm just joking... I'll cross it out!', but none of them ever asked me to follow through and cross out the extra words. On the contrary, with time, they began to dictate the same kinds of words themselves. What amazed me most was that the men too started ending their letters with expressions of affection and love. The women would often ask me, 'Did he really say that?' and exclaim, 'Read it again!' Sometimes I would read a sentence to them four times. I could see the happy glow in their eyes.

The letter-writing experience speaks volumes about the way a small risk, a different mindset, some personality and a little conversation can bring out something in people that they did not know they were missing. It shows how unexpected things can grow from the meeting of minds and ideas. I learned much in my early life about people, social relationships and behavioural change. I saw that in a complex and interconnected social system, if you can make one element work or behave differently, there is a good chance that other parts of the system will improve.

My father's advice to make my learning relevant to my people, and my own formative experiences and reflections as a letter writer, led me to a lifetime of involvement in community development and social research. As I returned to the village with my friends during school holidays, we looked for things to do when we were not working in the field. We started mobilising ourselves to provide sports and recreation activities such as table tennis and volleyball. These projects evolved into participation in much more complex community development initiatives related to schools, health clinics, potable water and roads. I found myself, increasingly and quite naturally, using what I later discovered to be participatory action research, a method of research that is grounded in the idea that lay people can become researchers in their own right. Communities of research can generate relevant knowledge to address the issues that are of priority concern to them. I was posing critical questions such as the following: What are we trying to do? Why are we doing it? Is there any evidence or precedent? What aspects are working and what aspects are not working so well? Who is benefiting and who is missing out? What needs to happen in order to improve the situation? How will we know if things are getting better? For a long time, I did not see any of these questions as research at all. This was just me and my attempts to make my education relevant to my community. After all, I was going to be a lawyer.

A turning point came when I completed my honours degree at the University of Ghana. The department invited me to become a tutor. The intention of my supervisors was that if I became a tutor, they could support me to secure a scholarship in order to study for a Doctor of Philosophy (PhD). That was the first time I considered the possibility of an academic career. My supervisors' plan came to fruition, and in 1982 I found myself at Glasgow University in Scotland, where despite the terrible weather (which is another story) I had an exciting, stimulating and fun time, both intellectually and socially. The main point is that I returned to the University of Ghana as an academic. At the same time, I began taking on more leadership positions in rural development projects in my village, such as the one I will now describe.

In 1986 there was a knock on my door early one morning. I opened the door and, to my surprise, saw two prominent leading elders from my village, Lieutenant Colonel Asamoah, or 'Colonel' as he was known, and Togbe Brusuo Letsu. 'What brings you here so early?' I wondered to myself. 'Has someone died at home?' I let them in and waited anxiously for what they had to say. 'We have come to talk to you about something that is important for Botoku', Colonel said. 'Togbe and I and our peers are getting old. We need younger people to take our place. We want you to use your education to help make Botoku a better place. We are asking you to become the Chairperson of the Botoku Electrification Committee. We want the committee to mobilise all Botoku people to give what they can according to their capacity. We want to make sure that Botoku is not left behind in the national rural electrification program'. It dawned on me then that I did not need to be a lawyer to make a real difference to people's lives. And so my role in community development leadership in the village began.

As an academic, I found myself embracing my community development involvement. I saw it as a real opportunity to engage communities of people in research, not only for their benefit but also for my own benefit in the form of publications and other academic outputs. Research, after all, is the creation of new knowledge or the use of existing knowledge to generate new understandings and ways of doing things. If I managed community development with the outlook of a researcher, then I could not only engage people in change, but build an evidence base as well. Research engagement is the process of facilitating the interaction between researchers and research users (such as policymakers, individuals and industry partners) for the mutually beneficial exchange of ideas and resources. Effective research engagement is the key to developing meaningful research questions and subsequently demonstrating research impact on society. Impact is the contribution, beyond academia, that research makes to an economy, society, environment or culture. In Ghana, I saw this working in the community development context. I worked on the development of physical infrastructure like schools, clinics and rural electrification, but, more importantly, I worked with communities to change entrenched cultural practices. Through these community development activities, cultural practices such as trial by ordeal for people accused of witchcraft and sorcery have been banned, even though belief in witchcraft and sorcery remains strong in Ghana.

I learned lessons from my Botoku community development work and from my close interactions with people like my father that, to this day, continue to influence the ways in which I seek to engage communities of people in research. Through my adventures as a letter writer, I learned that life is not so much about who you are or what you do but rather about the purpose and meaning that you attach to the things you do. You make your own meaning and your own work meaningful by matching your education and your efforts to the needs and aspirations of communities of people. Importantly, I also learned that no matter how desperate a community may look to an outsider, there are always pockets of strength, resilience and creativity. Small changes in social situations can have consequences far beyond what you may anticipate. It is the role of the researcher to find and work with these centres of strength and energy. One person can make a genuine difference.

Bibliography

Asamoah, F. M. K., & Tsey, K. (2012). *Botoku/Dzali: history, culture and governance. A learning resource for teachers, parents and students interested in African knowledge traditions.* Kwabenya, Accra: University Child and Youth Development Centre.

Australian Research Council. (2017a). Engagement and impact assessment pilot 2017. Report. Retrieved December 11, 2018, from http://www.arc.gov.au/sites/default/files/filedepot/Public/EI/Engagement_and_Impact_Assessment_Pilot_2017_Report.pdf.

Australian Research Council. (2017b). EI 2018 Submission guidelines. Retrieved December 11, 2018, from http://www.arc.gov.au/sites/default/files/filedepot/Public/EI/EI_2018_Submission_Guidelines.pdf.

Tsey, K. (2011). *Re-thinking development in Africa: An oral history approach from Botoku, Rural Ghana.* Cameroon: Langaa Research & Publishing Common Initiative Group.

Tsey, K., Patterson, D., Whiteside, M., Baird, L., & Baird, B. (2002). Indigenous men taking their rightful place in society? A preliminary analysis of a participatory action research process with Yarrabah Men's Health Group. *Australian Journal of Rural Health, 10,* 278–284. https://doi.org/10.1046/j.1440-1584.2002.00491.x.

Understanding the Context: The Case of Central Australian Aboriginal Health

2

Abstract

Research does not occur in a vacuum. It is important to develop an intellectual understanding of the social context of your research. Social researchers must listen to opinion leaders and synthesise academic literature, but they must also listen to the people they meet: children, the elderly, teenagers, men and women. Understanding the social context of your research requires curiosity; you must use everyday interactions and conversations with people as opportunities to learn. Your reading about history, politics, economics and the culture of a place should be as wide as possible. It is important to get a sense of the power dynamics at play in the dominant narratives. Ask whose voices are being shared and heard and whose are not. Who benefits from the status quo and who does not? How can things be made fairer? The tools and media available to analyse and understand social context of research will differ from place to place and over time. Source material may include journals, newspapers, textbooks, government or industry reports, social media, bulletin boards, conversations, literature reviews and even graffiti. This chapter illustrates my attempts to understand the social context of Central Australian Aboriginal health.

We have been trained to death ... we are the most trained group of people in this country but nothing has changed. We are still getting sick, our people are dying young, and we continue to rely on the goodwill of non-Aboriginal experts. We are still marking time. I'm sick of it all.

These were the first words I heard from a middle-level manager I was visiting to discuss the training needs of her organisation. I was new to Australia. I had just taken on a training coordinator role in Alice Springs, Central Australia, and the woman I was listening to worked for an Aboriginal community-controlled organisation. I was taken aback. I encouraged her to tell me more. She explained that almost all Aboriginal organisations had an *Aboriginalisation* policy. This policy was intended to assert Aboriginal self-determination and to nurture and support Aboriginal employees to gradually replace non-Aboriginal staff. My new client

© Springer Nature Switzerland AG 2019
K. Tsey, *Working on Wicked Problems*,
https://doi.org/10.1007/978-3-030-22325-0_2

called it the development of a 'culture of training'. For every non-Aboriginal employee, there had to be an Aboriginal trainee who would eventually take over that role. She did not see it as helpful. No Aboriginal people seemed to be taking the key jobs no matter how much training they had. The data backed up the woman's frustration. Over the years, most Aboriginal staff had undertaken some form of training, but they were not moving into the professional positions. Instead, a disturbing trend had emerged. As the organisations grew, new positions were created, and these positions became more technocratic, requiring higher levels of professional qualifications and skill. Invariably non-Aboriginal people filled these roles, and each new position spawned yet another Aboriginal co-worker. On paper, the organisation was growing, and more Aboriginal people were gaining employment, but the substantive professional positions were not filled by trained Aboriginal people because they lacked the recognised professional qualifications. My client asked, 'When are we going to stop being trainees and become normal employees like everyone else?' The basic question was: 'Why, after years of efforts to improve Aboriginal health, and encourage Aboriginal self-determination, was there no apparent change or improvement in their lives?'

As an outsider, I realised I needed to make sense of this situation. I needed to develop an understanding of what was happening in this country before I could make a place for myself as a researcher. It struck me that the news media at the time was full of references to Aboriginal health being a 'third-world' situation. The implication was that Aboriginal health could be viewed in a similar way to health in a developing nation. I wondered if the intention of the press was to stress the urgency or extent of Aboriginal disadvantage in health matters, but I questioned the comparison. I had the glimmer of an idea that, if I scrutinised this story through a different lens, I might gain a useful perspective. I had something the journalists lacked— genuine experience of a typical 'third-world' setting: my home country, Ghana. To aid my understanding, I decided to create a public dialogue around this third-world label drawing on my knowledge of public health policy developments in Ghana.

The task I set for myself was to unpack the meaning and implications associated with likening the Aboriginal health situation to third-world conditions. I consulted and researched widely, accessing statistical data as well as noting conversations I had with local people. I read up on history and consulted government health and economic data. I compared social and economic indicators for Ghana and the Central Australian Aboriginal population. I was concerned that the third-world label was being used as a convenient and grossly oversimplified way for politicians, the media and health professionals to divert attention away from identifying and addressing the true underlying causes of poor health among Aboriginal people. The numbers I collated for this exercise in the early 1990s were telling. I found two things that Ghanaians and Aboriginal Australians had in common—a life expectancy of 50–55 years and relatively high infant mortality. None of the other numbers, however, added up. The area in which the differences were greatest was health resources. Australia had far greater health resources than Ghana, supporting my initial misgivings about the validity of the comparison. In Ghana there was one doctor for every 23,000 people as opposed to one doctor for every 1200 people for

Central Australian Aboriginal people, a ratio 19 times better than Ghana's. Ghana spent $14 per person per year to provide health care for each of her 17 million people. Australia spent $600 per person (a conservative estimate) for Aboriginal people in Central Australia. This was half the amount Australia spent per head on the rest of the Australian population but more than 40 times the amount spent in Ghana.

In Ghana, access to health facilities for rural dwellers (who made up 70% of the population) was extremely limited. In fact, about 40% of people in Ghana at the time would never have seen a doctor in their lives. Traditional herbal and therapeutic spiritual healing would have been the only form of treatment they knew. Although Aboriginal people had more difficulty in accessing appropriate health services than the rest of the Australian population, the level of service in even the most remote of Australian communities was far better than that enjoyed by the majority of people in Ghana. In terms of income levels, Ghana and Australia were worlds apart. Ghana had an annual per capita gross national product (GNP) of $400. The equivalent figure for Australia was $17,000—although the average income for Aboriginal people was roughly half that of their non-Aboriginal counterparts. This meant that Aboriginal Australians had income levels roughly 30 times greater than people in Ghana, yet they shared a similar health status—obviously much lower than that of their non-Aboriginal counterparts. The key repeating information in these figures was that while Aboriginal people had access to better health resources than people in Ghana, they were generally much worse off than other Australians and had similar health outcomes to Ghanaians.

Like Australia, Ghana was once a British colony. Why were current patterns of health and social circumstances so different in these two countries? Why was the health of Aboriginal people, who enjoyed higher levels of medical care and income than people in Ghana, no better than that of Ghanaians? I looked to the history books. The British saw Ghana as a place to trade and exploit resources. As it was a crown colony (1874–1957), the British forced the local population to work on railway projects, build roads, work in mines and cut timber for exports. Africans were also encouraged into growing cocoa and other tropical crops for export. In Ghana, Indigenous labour formed the backbone of the colonial economy. In contrast, Australia was seen by the British primarily as a new homeland, a place to settle. Although Indigenous Australians often worked as unpaid domestic servants and cattlemen, their labour was never considered central to the settler economy. Indeed, the settlers saw the Indigenous population largely as a nuisance, to be killed or herded into institutions.

These different colonial philosophies and attitudes have affected modern Indigenous lifestyles. Traditionally, Ghanaians lived in small villages. The establishment of colonial administrative and commercial centres had resulted in urbanisation in Ghana, but the majority of Ghanaian people continued to live in their ancestral villages. In Australia, white settlement destroyed the traditional nomadic life. Settler policies demolished Indigenous forms of work without replacing them with work for wages. Uprooted and driven off their traditional lands, many Aboriginal Australians were forced together into artificially created church missions or government institutions or to the fringes of towns and cities. An important but often overlooked fact is that Aboriginal communities as we know them today were developed primarily as refugee camps for displaced people from numerous different cultural groups.

I discussed the differences between my native village and Central Australia with a friend and Aboriginal elder, Nagamara, a woman aged in her late 60s. During our conversation she asked me where I came from and whether alcohol was a problem in my community. She told me she was once a heavy drinker; she went days without food; she was very ill most of the time. She had thought that her death was only a matter of time and could not be bothered to look after herself. I asked how she had managed to get off alcohol. She remained silent for a while and then, with a smile, she said, 'Too many meetings and no time for grog'. Her move away from alcohol started when she was elected to represent her camp (because no one else was willing) on the board of management of the local health service. The more meetings she attended, the more she became interested in the affairs of the community. She was elected to the boards of the local housing association and language centre. She attended several meetings a week in addition to work with a night patrol, which was a group of community leaders and volunteers who patrolled the community to ensure intoxicated people were safe.

After hearing Nagamara's story, I explained why alcohol was not a major problem in my village at the time by describing a typical day in the life of my niece, Ama, an average Ghanaian rural dweller. Her day started at 5 am when she cooked black-eyed beans and plantain to sell to school children for breakfast. She attended to domestic chores, including fetching water from the stream, before leaving for the farm at 9 am with some breakfast for her husband. They grew cassava, yams, plantains, vegetables and spices. They also kept goats, sheep and chicken that were killed for special-occasion meals. Ama's working capital for cooking and selling breakfast was less than AU$30, but the income allowed her to earn money for items that the family did not produce, such as clothing, tools, fish and salt. Both Ama and her husband worked in their field until dusk when they returned to the village to prepare the evening meal for the family. After the children went to bed, Ama would spend another 2 h or so preparing food for cooking in the morning. This was her routine 6 days a week. Nagamara remained silent for some time, and then she said to me that there were two periods in her life when she felt healthy and in control of her life. One was when she had worked as a cook on a station; the work was difficult but it provided her a sense of purpose. The second time was her current community involvement.

Beyond health and living conditions, there were other key differences between growing up in rural Ghana and in an Indigenous community in Central Australia. In 1957, Ghana became independent. Although the economy was still heavily dependent on Britain and other industrialised nations, independence gave Ghanaians the opportunity to take their destiny into their own hands. In health matters, self-determination was popularly expressed through community development. Each village sets aside roughly 1 day in every 2 weeks for voluntary labour on community projects, including schools, health posts, roads, water projects and public toilets.

The government provided materials such as cement, roofing sheets and nails, while the community undertook the construction and maintenance of the infrastructure. In addition to the development of practical skills, there was generally a high degree of pride and sense of ownership of these community facilities. Education is another important part of the community development process. Communities in Ghana had no choice but to set up their own schools, train their own teachers and produce a critical mass of skilled people to run the economy from the village to the national level. In Australia, the political marginalisation of Aboriginal people is still demonstrated by the fact that there is no recognition of Indigenous people in the Australian Constitution.

Although Ghana and Indigenous Australia might learn from each other, it was clear to me that the different historical circumstances required different strategies for addressing health problems in the two societies. The one label of 'third-world conditions' was being used to describe two very different situations. I used this analysis to spark discussion and debate by way of a four-part piece in the local newspaper, the *Alice Springs News*. I learned early in my community development research career in Ghana that it was not enough to engage professionals through journal publications; one also needed to engage the broader community in public dialogues such as development forums, newspapers, radio and, in recent times, social media. I also produced an academic discussion paper to make the point that the lack of formal education was a significant barrier to improvements in Aboriginal health and self-determination.

There was an irony to my investigation. I was working as a training coordinator, seeking to bring positive health, education and other initiatives to Central Australia, but I had discovered that these initiatives were part of the problem. As mentioned at the beginning of this story, the bulk of employment being created by new initiatives was going to non-Aboriginal people who possessed the necessary formally recognised qualifications, skills and expertise. As a consequence, income inequality between the two population groups worsened. It was an unintended but nonetheless insidious effect that unhelpful role models and images were being created for Aboriginal children. In the health services, doctors, dentists, pharmacists and nurses were white, and Aboriginal health workers were black; in Aboriginal health research, researchers were predominantly white, and research assistants were black; in the schools, teachers were predominantly white, and teacher's aides were black. The list went on and on, begging the question: what type of role models were we creating for black children? The problem, however, was one I might also have the capacity to influence positively if I could make an impact in the education and training field.

Invaluable contributions were being made by health workers and other semi-professional Aboriginal people to their organisations and communities, but I could foresee the negative effects on young people of ethnically based career structures. Again, I compared my own experiences with those of Aboriginal Australian people. The first Aboriginal female lawyer in the Northern Territory, Lorraine Liddle, tells the story of how, as a student, she told her high school career counsellor she wanted to become a lawyer and was told this was a ridiculous dream. Lorraine had never met an Aboriginal lawyer at the time, and this helped to convince her that as an

Aboriginal girl she could not expect to follow that path. So she trained as a teacher instead. Years later, she visited Papua New Guinea and, for the first time, realised that black people could be lawyers or doctors or accountants. In contrast, my own childhood dream to become a lawyer, as described in Chap. 1, was made at my primary school in rural Ghana in a world where all the lawyers, doctors and teachers I knew were black.

It was simply not true to argue that Aboriginal health was poor because they lived in third-world conditions. Furthermore, this type of simplistic reasoning could be dangerous since it masked or drew attention away from the real cause of Aboriginal ill health: the markedly inferior position in social class, including the lack of influence or power that Aboriginal people, as a group, held relative to the rest of Australian society. Indigenous Australians have always known that improvements in their health depended on having greater control over their lives and the things that affected them. This places responsibility not only on the governments but on the wider society, to create an environment where Indigenous people feel they are a legitimate part of society and can participate at all levels on their own terms. Better education and employment opportunities are key to such participation. Equally important is the creation of appropriate channels that would allow Indigenous people to have genuine influence over government policies and programs that affect them. (My argument at that time in many ways foreshadowed the current calls for constitutional recognition for Indigenous Australians.)

The problems that I sought to understand and contextualise have no straightforward solutions. Researchers, like society, are increasingly engaged with issues that are best described as *wicked problems*. At the core of wicked problems is the challenge of sustainability. In a world of finite resources, how should we as humans live our lives in ways that do not disadvantage others within present or future generations? Communities, workplaces and families are transforming in complex and rapid ways into the future. The past is catching up with communities too. The hurt and trauma of dispossession, racism and colonialism have left a mark on new generations. The world today is very different from that of the early 1990s when I embarked on this meaning-making exercise to better understand the Central Australian Aboriginal social health situation. Some of the media pieces which formed the basis of this chapter, for example, were written using a typewriter; a researcher going through a similar exercise today will likely be using the Internet for their research and social media as a key engagement tool in sharing their insights. Nevertheless, the challenge of understanding the nature of the underlying causes of the social health gap between Indigenous and other Australians remains, sadly, as relevant today as it was nearly 30 years ago. The remaining stories in this book show my attempts to inform my research engagement by using my understanding of the importance of education, self-determination, empowerment and control over destiny as critical factors in enabling communities of people to improve their own health and wellbeing.

Bibliography

Chryssides, H. (1993). *Local heroes*. Melbourne: Collins Dove.

Devitt, J., Hall, G., & Tsey, K. (2001a). Underlying causes. In J. Condon, G. Warman, & L. Arnold (Eds.), *The health and welfare of Territorians* (pp. 9–18). Darwin: Territory Health Services.

Devitt, J., Hall, G., & Tsey, K. (2001b). *An introduction to the social determinants of health in relation to the Northern Territory Indigenous population* (pp. 1–20). Darwin: CRC for Aboriginal & Tropical Health.

Guy Peters, B. (2017). What is so wicked about wicked problems? A conceptual analysis and research program. *Policy and Society, 36*(3), 385–396.

Tsey, K. (1994a, May 12). Black health: The third world myth. *Alice Springs News*, p. 1.

Tsey, K. (1994b, May 19). Aboriginal health: How others cope. *Alice Springs News*, p. 2.

Tsey, K. (1994c, May 26). How British ambition shaped two different black destinies: Colonialism and indigenous health in Ghana and Australia. *Alice Springs News*, p. 2.

Tsey, K. (1994d, April 3). Health and independence: How effective is indigenous self determination in Ghana and Australia? *Alice Springs News*, p. 2.

Tsey, K. (1996). Aboriginal self-determination, education and health: Towards a more radical attitude towards Aboriginal education. In *Proceedings of the Aboriginal health cultural transitions conference, Northern Territory University, Darwin, 28–30 September 1995* (pp. 178–186). Darwin: NTU Press.

Tsey, K. (1997). Aboriginal self-determination, education and health: Towards a more radical attitude towards Aboriginal education. *Australian and New Zealand Journal of Public Health, 21*(1), 77–83.

Tsey, K. (1999, February 3). Five years on: What we gained and lost in Aboriginal health. *Alice Springs News*, p. 3.

Wilkinson, R., & Marmot, M. (1998). *Social determinants of health: The solid facts*. Copenhagen: WHO Regional Office for Europe.

Learning by Doing: Community Action Against Sex, Alcohol and Violence in Tennant Creek

3

Abstract

As a social researcher, it is highly likely that you will need to accept your vulnerability when throwing yourself, often personally as well as professionally, into the deep end of a difficult problem for which there is no easy solution in sight. Problems such as this chapter describes, the use of sex to promote alcohol sales in an Aboriginal community and the consequent interpersonal violence, can seem insurmountable. Working on these types of problems, wicked problems, means having the understanding that one researcher, no matter how wonderful their ideas, will not have all the answers. Researchers are more effective if they take a collaborative learn-by-doing approach, thereby building confidence that research partners and researchers are in it together. Each individual, organisation, group and researcher brings specific expertise to a project, and through collaborative approaches, problems can be worked around as they appear.

The Northern Territory town of Tennant Creek—once the epicentre of a gold-mining boom—has a long (and ongoing) history of tragedy, trouble and sex-related violence on the one hand and resilience of the local Aboriginal people and their community organisations on the other. Tennant Creek was one of the first Australian towns in which I engaged in research and community development after I left Ghana. It was also the place where I realised the potential and importance of taking a collaborative learn-by-doing approach to social and community development-based research engagement and impact. In a collaborative learn-by-doing model, researcher and research community learn from one another. The research community shares its perspectives, ideas and data. The researchers share their expertise about data collection, organisation, research planning, analysis, presentation of research findings and demonstration of impact. If conducted in a truly collaborative way, the process of analysing, synthesising and presenting research data into research findings is, in itself, a form of capacity building and

© Springer Nature Switzerland AG 2019
K. Tsey, *Working on Wicked Problems*,
https://doi.org/10.1007/978-3-030-22325-0_3

community development. Health workers, community members and leaders who participate in this process of synthesising data become novice researchers. They gain the foundations, skills and insights that are necessary for they themselves to become researchers or know how to facilitate and plan for research impact. The story I tell here, set against a backdrop of alcohol-fuelled sex tourism and violence in a remote Northern Australian town, illustrates the way social researchers can work with community and professional groups to add another dimension—a research dimension—to their work.

In the early 1990s, I attended a conference in Alice Springs where I delivered a slide presentation on community development in rural Ghana. Among those who came to listen to my talk were two people from Tennant Creek. The pair approached me and asked whether it would be possible for me to join them in Tennant Creek at the end of the conference in 2 days' time. They thought that Tennant Creek Aboriginal people might be interested in the things I discussed in my talk. I had been in Australia (based in the city of Sydney) for only 6 months and was struggling to make sense of the situation in Indigenous communities; I was curious to meet the people working at the coalface and keen to learn from them. So, without really knowing what I was getting myself into, I said yes.

The country of Ghana is the size of the state of Victoria in Australia but has the same population as the whole of Australia. In Ghana, where population density is relatively high, you cannot travel for 20 km without coming to another village or town. The roads are poor and even a 100 km trip must be well-planned; it can take half a day to drive this distance. So when my hosts told me that Tennant Creek was the next town north of Alice Springs, I thought it would be a drive of an hour or less. Australia's roads seemed good compared with Ghana's. The next town could not be too far away. Little did I know, we would be embarking on a 500 km drive on a highway that, at the time, had no speed limit. After about 4 h of driving—an indication of how fast we travelled the distance—we arrived in Tennant Creek. I was shown around the health service, met health workers and board members and visited the dam and the Aboriginal sacred pebble site. It was then time for my slide show, which was attended by about 25 people. The audience was particularly interested in the Ghanaian model of rural development partnerships. These partnerships were between the non-resident villagers who had left for employment and education opportunities and the residents remaining in the village. Non-residents contributed technical expertise and finance, while residents, with government support, provided manual labour to build schools, clinics, markets and roads. While some Tennant Creek people said they felt lucky to be in Australia, where people didn't need to do hard labour just to build two or three small classroom blocks, others commented that it might not be a bad thing for people to work hard to build facilities. They believed people would be more likely to value them and less likely to damage or vandalise them, as was apparently common in Tennant Creek at the time.

The following day my hosts gave me a presentation describing the range of services and projects in which the health service was involved. One major initiative in which I became involved was a community action, led by the Aboriginal community-controlled health service, to put a stop to local pubs using striptease shows to promote the sale of alcohol. Tennant Creek was originally a mining town. Legend has it that a truck carrying beer from Adelaide to Darwin in the late nineteenth century broke down along the journey, and the driver and the support crew settled down and started drinking the cargo; the place where the beer truck broke down became Tennant Creek. The official history is a little different from the local legend. In its gold-mining heyday, Tennant Creek had a population of 5000 and many alcohol outlets. In the mid-1980s the gold mines closed and thousands of residents moved on. The population almost halved, sparking intense competition among the pubs for the diminishing number of patrons. The pubs decided to reinvent themselves, and, almost overnight, Tennant Creek was turned into an exotic striptease oasis in the semi-desert. Young women were imported from around the country to perform from Thursday lunchtime to Sunday night. Men came from the neighbouring cattle stations, from Alice Springs, Darwin, Perth and all over Australia to witness these sex shows. In their efforts to outdo each other, pubs reduced the price of alcohol to ridiculously low levels during happy hour shows.

The local health service was the first to object to the use of striptease to promote alcohol sales. The doctors and health workers believed they were seeing more alcohol-related assaults and injuries in the clinic, which they attributed to the availability of cheap alcohol. At the time of the community action, the Northern Territory had the highest alcohol consumption per capita in Australia and the highest number of licenced outlets. Research had already showed strong links between alcohol availability, alcohol consumption and alcohol-related harm. In the late 1980s, Alice Springs had more than 70 retail liquor outlets, approximately one for every 330 people, and Tennant Creek had 14 outlets or 1 for every 215 people. The emphasis on drinking in the Northern Territory was embedded in popular culture. For instance, there was the idea in the Territory that the size of a town could be measured by the number of its pubs, and the lyrics of folk musician and Territorian, Ted Egan, boasted: 'We've got some bloody good drinkers in the Northern Territory'.

For the 9 months before my visit to Tennant Creek, my hosts, together with the health service, had been leading a community campaign to stop the striptease shows and happy hours. The community was sharply divided into pro-striptease show and anti-striptease show camps. The health service representatives in Tennant Creek kept meticulous records of the campaign. The records included minutes of public meetings, attended by up to 50 people, extensive newspaper coverage by both local and national papers and recordings from radio and TV programs. My first question was whether anyone had been analysing the information in the form of action research. When they said no, I told them that, from a participatory research point of view, they were sitting on their own gold mine. It was important for a person with the relevant skills and expertise to collate and analyse the accumulating information as transparently as possible.

The analysis could be presented at community meetings for the attention of both the pro- and anti-striptease camps. I said that, done properly, the results of the research could serve as a mirror for both sides to reflect on their attitudes and beliefs regarding the conflict. An effective analysis could move the process past the conflict and arguments that had become the focus of the issue and lead to progress. By compiling and analysing the information at hand, an artefact could be produced that contained irrefutable evidence and deeper insight. Change could be sparked if this artefact was shared with the right people through the right channels. As a social researcher and community development advocate, I could see how I could use my skills to help. I pointed out to my hosts: 'You brought me all the way from Alice Springs to tell you about community development. But this is community development you are doing. The only difference is that I research and write about mine, and you are not analysing and writing about yours'. I could see quite clearly the way I could, as a researcher, document and highlight the incremental achievements and challenges in ways that enabled further action.

Before I left Tennant Creek, we made plans for my return: a longer stay during which I could facilitate and write up an analysis of the community action. Poring through the data was a fascinating and troubling exercise. The first rumblings against the striptease shows developed within Tennant Creek's Aboriginal community. There were two main drivers for the opposition. Firstly, the main hotels that embraced and promoted the striptease shows had traditionally been places where Aboriginal people gathered and drank. For some Aboriginal patrons and families, the shows were seen as an unwarranted intrusion and, given the high level of alcohol abuse in the Aboriginal community, an exploitation of their drinking habits. Aboriginal people felt targeted. Secondly, there was a growing awareness within the health service and the wider community of a clear link between the striptease shows, alcohol consumption and violence, especially towards women and children. On one occasion a 15-year-old youth who attended a show was convicted of sexually assaulting a 40-year-old woman on his way home from that show. The judge did not draw a link between the show and the assault in the courtroom, but the community wondered aloud about cause and effect. In another instance, a young woman who apparently exposed herself during an audience participation competition was raped on her way home by a man who had been at the show. As a primary health care organisation, the health service had followed up the care of these victims with community action to address the broader social, economic and political causes of this violence.

The Aboriginal community also expressed concerns that the combination of sex and alcohol would further expose the community to the dangers of sexually transmitted diseases, including human immunodeficiency virus (HIV), because of the growing culture of irresponsible and unprotected sex. A related concern of the Aboriginal community was the violation of their cultural values, that striptease shows were 'not our way', as expressed by an elder, Topsy Nelson, on the Australian Broadcasting Corporation (ABC) 7.30 Report. The non-Aboriginal community, particularly women, were also concerned about the shows. Many women saw the shows as pornography that degraded and exploited women, reinforcing an unhealthy attitude of objectification and male dominance over submissive females.

The anti-striptease lobby had looked beyond their town for support and assistance. They had developed an extensive system of networking throughout the Northern Territory. Their supporters included the Women's Information Centre in Darwin, Campaign Against Sexual Exploitation (CASE), the Prostitutes' Collective based in Darwin, the Ruby-Gaea Darwin Centre Against Rape, government agencies and churches. Tennant Creek meeting resolutions, which were recorded methodically, were circulated widely among supporters, and these supporter groups constantly lobbied Territory politicians on behalf of Tennant Creek people. Support for the anti-striptease lobby was so strong that in January 1989 a public meeting was held in Darwin, some 980 km away, in support of the Tennant Creek action.

Although the pro-striptease lobby was a smaller group, it had significant economic and political clout. Their strategies to counteract the opposition to the shows included arguments such as the shows were harmless, people in the community wanted them and individuals had the right to attend if they wanted. Other strategies and arguments included the dismissal of the anti-striptease lobby as emotional, sensational or 'wowsers', a colloquial Australian word that describes an excessively puritanical person. They tried to make the anti-striptease position appear extreme by claiming that the community action was aimed at outlawing striptease and prostitution altogether. In fact, the anti-striptease lobby was calling for more regulation and legalisation of the sex industry, as demanded by the Darwin Prostitutes' Collective. The pro-striptease lobby also encouraged strippers to argue that they were being victimised for doing their job. As one stripper later put it to the media: 'They [the wowsers] think we get out there and we provoke these men into a sexual frenzy and they have to take it out on somebody. It's a load of crap'. The pro-striptease camp also resorted to intimidation. Two bouncers were threatened with legal action after they provided affidavits to the anti-striptease lobby claiming that prostitution was occurring at the hotel after the shows. Intimidation did not stop at threats. Husbands, boyfriends and other male striptease-show sympathisers reportedly used violence to harass and physically prevent women from attending the public meetings.

The debate attracted the attention of local and national media and politicians. The stories made sensational newspaper headlines: 'Lust in the dust'; 'Up the creek without a stitch'; 'Tennant meets over stripper outrage'; 'Secrets of strip show patrons'; 'No show, pro show', 'Wife bashers ball'; 'White fella wank'; and 'Women on rampage'. Although some of the headlines were vulgar and shocking, a significant proportion of the stories were written by female journalists sympathetic to the anti-striptease cause. Their willingness to throw their weight behind the anti-striptease lobby against powerful interest groups contributed to the success of the community action. The local Aboriginal community-controlled health service had brought together a diverse group of individuals and interest groups from all sections of the community and beyond. They had generated an enormous amount of data that spoke directly to the importance of community mobilisation in effecting social change. I sat down with key members of the lobby team, and, together, we turned their activism and record-keeping into research findings.

The experience of co-writing this paper with practitioners working at the coalface brought home to me the need to engage the Indigenous community-controlled sector as a critical first step in doing research that addresses the needs and aspirations of Indigenous people. The publication of our paper marked an important first step in this direction. By taking advantage of my chance encounter with the Tennant Creek people who later became my co-authors, John Boffa and Chris George, I was able to demonstrate how a collaborative learn-by-doing approach to research might help Aboriginal organisations to build healthier communities and share their stories with others. Together, we worked to our strengths. The health service used their public health knowledge and record-keeping skills. Community groups supported lobbying action. And I used my skills as a researcher to progress the issue to resolution and follow-on community action. The paper that came out of this collaboration, 'Sex, alcohol and violence: a community action against the use of strip tease to promote the sale of alcohol', published in the *Australian and New Zealand Journal of Public Health*, was awarded the Australian Public Health Association's JM Thompson Award for good practice in public health. This was my first publication in Aboriginal health.

The sustained community action to curb sex tourism, alcohol abuse and violence in Tennant Creek led to real social change. The campaign opened the door to changes to the Northern Territory *Liquor Act* which turned a previously voluntary code of ethics into law. The new law made it compulsory for licensees to warn the public that striptease shows were on, to conduct the shows behind closed doors, not to allow any audience participation and to keep a specified distance between the strippers and the audience. In this new, safer format, the shows failed to attract the same numbers of patrons and soon ceased altogether, returning only occasionally, modified in accordance with the new guidelines and staged under police and community vigilance. The community action also contributed to the establishment of a women's refuge, the resourcing of Aboriginal organisations to develop alcohol intervention and rehabilitation programs and the promotion of sports and recreation activities.

Bibliography

Australian Broadcasting Corporation. (1989, April 23). *7.30 report*. Darwin: ABC.

Boffa, J., George, C., & Tsey, K. (1994). Sex, alcohol and violence: A community collaborative action against strip tease shows. *Australian Journal of Public Health, 18*(4), 359–366.

Boffa, J., George, C., & Tsey, K. (1995). Sex, alcohol and violence: a community collaborative action against strip tease shows. In J. Richters & R. Pike (Eds.), *Public health practice in Australia: winning entries for the Medibank Private J. Ashburton Thompson Award for Public Health Practice 1994*. Canberra: Public Health Association of Australia Inc..

Building Capacity for Research: The Lowitja Institute

4

Abstract

For social research to be meaningful for Indigenous Australians and, for that matter, any community of people, the intended beneficiaries of the research must be in the driver's seat. Informed consent is simply not enough in social research. The research community must be involved in formulating the research questions as well as finding answers. To make this possible, social researchers need to get involved in building research capacity as a core component of their projects. Communities must be resourced and supported to develop the capability to do their own research, set their own priorities and make informed decisions about research that affects them. This type of capacity development may include funding, mentoring, training, scholarships, awards and placements for individual people from the research community. It may also involve creating systems, processes and capabilities in community organisations whose core business is not research. It is also important that communities have control and a real say in the funding for research. This story about the development of the Lowitja Institute and its predecessors, the Cooperative Research Centres for Indigenous health, illustrates the importance of agency, capacity and community control in terms of Aboriginal and Torres Strait Islander health research.

When I began working with Aboriginal people in Central Australia as a researcher, the relationship between researchers, Aboriginal organisations and community leaders was extremely volatile. Trust was non-existent. The Aboriginal people felt they had been 'researched to death without anything to show for it'. The university-based researchers believed there were important research questions to be answered and that their findings could be used to make improvements, but their primary focus often was to get PhDs, publications or promotions. The prevailing research approach might best be described as 'fly-in, fly-out', much like workers at a remote mine. Very few Aboriginal people in the communities were conducting their own research, and very

© Springer Nature Switzerland AG 2019
K. Tsey, *Working on Wicked Problems*,
https://doi.org/10.1007/978-3-030-22325-0_4

few researchers I met in the universities were Aboriginal people. Meaningful conversations between Aboriginal people and researchers were few and far between. These two groups were quite different and discrete. This gap in communication and goals, incidentally, is not unique to this sphere of research; I have seen researchers working in many different areas of the community who just do not know how to engage with community or industry (or even that they need to) and vice versa.

Against this background of a seemingly unbridgeable gap between researchers and Aboriginal organisations, I was invited to join a proposed Cooperative Research Centre (CRC) for Aboriginal and Tropical Health. I jumped at the opportunity with alacrity, seeing it as a way to work as part of a team that could try to get researchers to engage more effectively with Aboriginal organisations. I was in a slightly different situation from most researchers at the time. I had not come straight to research, having spent more than 2 years working with Aboriginal organisations to train health workers, managers and program coordinators about how to plan, implement and evaluate community programs. I was not, therefore, a typical university researcher whose primary work was entirely removed from the day-to-day Aboriginal experience. Working in Aboriginal organisations had allowed me to develop important relationships with key individuals, and I was routinely invited to evaluate programs and services.

The CRC scheme had been introduced as a way of getting researchers and industry to work more collaboratively and productively so that industry might inform research and research, in turn, could inform industry. This was a very tangible move towards the concept that research must have impact that extends beyond the confines of academia. It was recognised that it takes time and requires continuity of commitment to make a lasting impact. So, unlike the usual 2- to 3-year duration of research grants, CRCs were to be funded for up to 7 years with an opportunity, subject to productivity, to renew for an additional 7 years. All CRC partners had to contribute financially and in-kind to demonstrate their investment in and commitment to the proposed research. The Menzies School of Health Research, with whom I was working at the time, had made an application to lead a CRC in the past but had not been successful, seemingly because there was insufficient Aboriginal support for their proposal. The Menzies director was anxious to ensure that he 'did the right thing this time, by Aboriginal people'.

As one of five program leaders in the proposed CRC (with responsibility for the education and health program area), I was required to visit Aboriginal health services, education providers and other organisations to talk with them generally about the proposed CRC and about the education and health program in particular. I had meetings with individuals and small groups and held workshops in Alice Springs and Darwin. I used a snowballing technique whereby I treated each meeting or workshop as an opportunity to point me in the next direction or set up another meeting with a stakeholder. For the 6 months leading up to the application deadline, I devoted an average of 1 or 2 days a week to the consultations.

Several things stood out for me from the outset. Firstly, researchers with university ethics approval could no longer simply go into Indigenous communities and do whatever research they wanted. From the late 1980s, Aboriginal community-controlled health services had taken the lead in insisting that they must have a real say in the research that was being done in Aboriginal communities. They wanted to ensure that the research was of benefit to the communities. In theory, a good thing, but in practise, something else. While Aboriginal health services were committed to having a genuine say in what went on in Aboriginal health research, the reality was, and still is, that they are not research organisations. Their purpose is to provide health services in communities suffering some of the highest burdens of disease. The entire culture of these organisations revolves around providing health care, not carrying out research.

Once Aboriginal organisations decided to have a say in determining research agendas as part of their general struggle for self-determination, it became a requirement of the National Health and Medical Research Council (NHMRC) and other funding bodies that any researcher proposing to do Aboriginal health research must first secure the support of the relevant Aboriginal community organisation. Most of these health services and communities were not resourced sufficiently, nor did they have the required expertise, to make informed decisions on the usefulness or otherwise of research proposals. Consequently, Aboriginal health organisations either dragged their feet regarding requests for research support letters or managers simply rubber-stamped proposals to satisfy researchers anxious about missing tight funding deadlines.

Aboriginal health service managers suggested from the start that if researchers genuinely wanted to work with them on research, then it was imperative that their health organisations were resourced to develop the understanding and capacity to make informed decisions about research priorities. From my point of view, a commitment to fund dedicated research positions within these Aboriginal health service and CRC partner organisations was a turning point in building confidence among Aboriginal health leaders. The positions, which came to be known as Aboriginal Medical Services Research Fellows, were the first positions to be recruited once a CRC was funded. Another defining feature of the proposed CRC, which further signalled the willingness of researchers to work in partnership with Aboriginal people, was the decision to staff the CRC governing body with an Indigenous majority and an Indigenous chairperson.

One major concern, frequently raised, was how to ensure that the new CRC did not become yet another avenue for non-Indigenous researchers to further their academic ambitions at the expense of Indigenous people. A senior manager from an Indigenous organisation repeatedly asked throughout the different stages of the consultation: 'This is what I want to know ... what exactly is in it for my organisation? How will it benefit my people?' Throughout the consultations, Indigenous participants, especially those working in education, repeatedly told me that they would participate only as principal researchers in their own right and not simply as research assistants or support workers. An Indigenous educator made another point: 'Aboriginal organisations have tried hard to do their own research ... but even when we succeed in getting the money to do the research, we still have to employ non-Aboriginal people as the principal researchers ... the research belongs to the organisation but in the end they [non-Indigenous researchers] continue to be the experts in the field ... what I'm saying is some of us know the power of research and we [Indigenous people] want to become principal researchers too'.

There was a widespread perception that Indigenous people suffered from what one person called 'consultation fatigue'. In the absence of coordinated approaches from the many different agencies that were involved in research in Indigenous communities, there was a systematic failure to follow-up to ensure that research recommendations were acted on appropriately. Some people feared that a major initiative such as the proposed CRC might escalate consultation fatigue without significant benefits to the participating communities. Such attitudes were reinforced by the view that researchers were only skilled in describing and analysing problems, when the priority for most Indigenous people was how to solve the problems and implement solutions: 'Researchers are good at saying what the problem is ... what we want to know is how to keep our children at school, so they can grow up and feel good about themselves'.

Menzies' bid to establish a Cooperative Research Centre for Aboriginal Tropical Health (CRCATH) was ultimately successful and would evolve over the years as priorities and funding arrangements changed. Following the formal inauguration of CRCATH in July 1997, a reference group chaired by a veteran Aboriginal educator, Professor Paul Hughes from Flinders University in Adelaide, was set up to provide support and strategic direction for the education and health research program. A major outcome of the preliminary consultation was the identification of what amounted to a shopping list of over a dozen possible research and development ideas related to health and education. Two Research Fellows were employed to undertake the program review, further the community consultation process and assist in developing the medium- to long-term research strategy.

As a result of the program review, two parallel action research projects were designed and funded to explore the relationships between education and health in the context of Indigenous people in the northern (Top End) and southern (Central Australia) halves of the Northern Territory. An important feature of the two projects was that they were both specifically designed around teams of local Indigenous educators, researchers and trainee researchers, supported by non-Indigenous researchers as partners and mentors. The rationale was to enhance local Indigenous research capacity as a necessary first step in effective Indigenous participation in the research agenda. While the research findings were important, the process of supporting Indigenous people to develop an understanding of research and to make informed decisions about research relating to Indigenous communities was seen as an end in itself.

There were two major outcomes from the education-health program of research with longer-term implications for Indigenous health research. Firstly, there was rapid accumulation of a body of knowledge exploring the relationships between education and health in the context of Indigenous Australians. All reports acknowledged the importance of education for Indigenous children, although the associations with health were found to be inconclusive or less straightforward. The reports also identified a range of barriers as well as strategies to improve Indigenous education outcomes.

The other major outcome was research capacity building. Not only did we enable, train and support Indigenous researchers involved in the projects, but we also built skills and goodwill in the communities themselves. For example, the eight Indigenous researchers employed within one of the education-health projects reported that, despite creating a steep learning curve for themselves, the participatory approach to the research meant that the community had become more familiar with the positive aspects of a Western research culture. 'This sort of participatory research should be supported in the community. This is how research should be done, starting something for the community and not just taking the information away ... in the past nothing happened from research. This is the first time that research from the outside has collected information for the community. It is a different way'.

Since then, the concept of enhancing the capacity of Indigenous people to participate in research has come a long way. Key Indigenous research leaders within the CRC, including Professor Ian Anderson, then CRC director of research, advocated for dedicated NHMRC funding for building Indigenous research capacity. Between the early 2000s and 2014, the NHMRC awarded a total of ten capacity-building grants to teams of Indigenous researchers, supported by experienced Indigenous or non-Indigenous researchers. In 2007, I was part of a James Cook University (JCU) team that won a $2.5 million, 5-year grant to mentor and support 20 early career Indigenous researchers to attain research higher degrees and other research expertise.

The CRCATH itself became the Cooperative Research Centre for Aboriginal and Torres Strait Islander Health (2003–2009) and subsequently, since 2010, the Lowitja Institute—Australia's only national Indigenous-controlled health research organisation. All three organisations have maintained a particular focus over the years on collaboration, knowledge exchange and ensuring that research is translated into improved services for Indigenous people. The original Indigenous 'Education and Health' program of research (1997–2003), which was the focus of my formative consultation, morphed firstly into the 'Social Determinants of Health' program of research during the second CRC for Aboriginal Health (2004–2009) and then the 'Social and Emotional Wellbeing' program when the third CRC became the Lowitja Institute in 2010.

In 2012, the chairperson of the Lowitja Institute, Pat Anderson, reflected on the many changes since 1997. She recalled that at the first CRCATH planning workshop in Darwin in 1997, researchers were in one corner of the room and Indigenous people and other service providers were in the other corner. She had needed to facilitate discussion between the groups. By the afternoon of that day, a few of the researchers left frustrated, but many continued and are still involved today. Now she sees many Indigenous and non-Indigenous people—researchers, service providers and community members—sharing ideas and information about how to improve Indigenous health. After years of collaborating personally with the various CRCs and the Lowitja Institute, it is gratifying, to say the least, to look back and appreciate how far researchers, both Indigenous and non-Indigenous, have come in their efforts to create meaningful professional relationships and engage with mutual respect with Indigenous service providers and communities. This has become evident at Lowitja Institute conferences, knowledge-sharing forums and other research translation events over the years. It is sad, however, that after more than 20 years, the Lowitja

Institute is yet to secure ongoing Commonwealth funding to protect and extend the gains of collaborative research in such vital niche areas as the uptake of research evidence into practise.

For research to truly address the needs and aspirations of Indigenous Australians, the importance of research capacity must be recognised, not just at the level of individual researchers, but also at an institutional level, such as with the Lowitja Institute. There is an urgent need for the NHMRC, the Commonwealth Department of Health and the Lowitja Institute to work together to consider sustainable funding models whereby a dedicated proportion of the core national health research funding is quarantined for and administered by the Lowitja Institute. For me personally, the Lowitja Institute and its predecessor CRCs provided the supportive environments that allowed me, as a member of several different teams, to undertake collaborative empowerment and wellbeing research with many Indigenous organisations and communities across Australia, as Chaps. 5–8 illustrate.

Bibliography

Australian Institute of Aboriginal and Torres Strait Islander Studies & The Lowitja Institute. (2017). *Changing the narrative in Aboriginal and Torres Strait islander health research: Four cooperative research centres and the Lowitja Institute: The story so far*. Melbourne: The Lowitja Institute.

Boughton, B. (2000). What is the connection between Aboriginal education and Aboriginal health? In *Cooperative Research Centre for Aboriginal & Tropical Health (CRCATH) occasional papers series, 2*. Darwin: CRCATH.

Katona, M., Cahil, R., Wumpa, E., Biritjalawuy, B., & Lowell, A. (2000). *Indigenous health and education: Exploring the connections: A CRC research report*. Darwin: Cooperative Research Centre for Aboriginal & Tropical Health.

Malin, M. (2003). Is schooling good for Aboriginal children? In *Cooperative Research Centre for Aboriginal & Tropical Health (CRCATH) occasional papers series, 8*. Darwin: CRCATH.

Thomas, D. P., Bainbridge, R., & Tsey, K. (2014). Changing discourses in Aboriginal and Torres Strait Islander health research, 1914–2014. *Medical Journal of Australia, 201*, S1–S4. https://doi.org/10.5694/mja14.00114.

Tsey, K. (2001). Making research more relevant to the needs and aspirations of indigenous Australians: The importance of research capacity development. *Aboriginal and Islander Health Worker Journal, 25*(1), 19–24.

Developing Self-Awareness as a Researcher: The Family Wellbeing Program

5

Abstract

As a researcher, you have ideas and assumptions about how to bring about change in a social situation. These ideas are built upon a firm (and privileged) base whose main feature is access to both information and knowledge. When dealing with wicked problems and complex issues, such as how to prevent suicide among Indigenous youth, you must learn to put some ideas aside and support the research community to be the drivers of their own change. The social researcher becomes, in large part, a critical friend. Trust and knowledge must be built as the process unfolds. In this chapter, I introduce a program I encountered early in my Australian academic career, the Aboriginal Family Wellbeing program. This program, developed by an Aboriginal community in South Australia, has become an enduring feature of the work I do to assist communities to build their own capacity for change. In recent years, I have come to realise that this model, which is based on Indigenous research principles, has deep and abiding potential to build capacity, including self-awareness and positive mindset, not just in research communities, but also in researchers themselves.

In the early days of my research career, I believed that social change occurred only through collective action, either explicit or implicit, directed at changing the oppressive structures and institutions of society. On moving to Australia, I discovered that this belief was lacking in depth, in part because it failed to take into account an important human element. This realisation was triggered by my exposure in Alice Springs to a program called the Aboriginal Family Wellbeing (FWB) empowerment program and required me to address some personal biases. The program was developed as a tool to engage and enable individuals and communities to take greater control over and responsibility for their own social health. The tool, however, is also relevant and effective in helping researchers themselves. In this chapter, I

© Springer Nature Switzerland AG 2019
K. Tsey, *Working on Wicked Problems*,
https://doi.org/10.1007/978-3-030-22325-0_5

explain my introduction to the Aboriginal Family Wellbeing empowerment program and my subsequent enduring research relationship with it.

I first encountered the FWB program in Alice Springs when I was asked to evaluate its effectiveness. FWB had been trialled in Alice Springs in response to the growing suicide rates of young men in the town. The human tragedy of these deaths was occurring at a time when the Alice Springs community itself was at the forefront of an empowerment movement that had led to greater self-determination; this made the terrible occurrences of the suicides even more bewildering. Alice Springs had, after more than 30 years of struggle by Aboriginal leaders and activists, accrued a long list of milestones and achievements. They had developed community-controlled organisations. They had established a Land Council. They had an Aboriginal legal service, a comprehensive primary health-care service, a media company, a housing organisation, a centre for appropriate technology, a women's council, a tertiary training institute and a primary school teaching children in four Aboriginal languages as well as in English. Yet this community was seeing its young people, the very generation they were fighting for, taking their own lives for reasons no one could understand. There was an overwhelming sense of urgency.

During discussions about suicide in the community, one man had proposed a program organised by Aboriginal people in South Australia called Family Wellbeing. The program was developed to give Aboriginal people the capabilities to deal with the day-to-day problems they faced living as a minority Indigenous culture within mainstream Australia. He had said that FWB helped people to reflect on questions such as: Who am I? What are my basic physical, emotional, mental and spiritual needs? Are these needs being met? What about those needs of my family, friends and community? What can I do to ensure my needs and those of my family are appropriately met? The program sought to help or empower people to participate in work and education and to be the parents they wanted to be. It was to be my task to evaluate the delivery and impact of the program.

I initially felt a degree of cynicism about the program. As someone who was generally sceptical of 'new-age' approaches, I felt misgivings and uncertainty when I was faced with terms such as *healing, inner qualities, heart-centred* and *visualisation* throughout the course material I reviewed. A program that wanted to teach individuals how to 'feel good about themselves and with each other', without explicitly tackling the underlying structural causes of inequality in society, struck me as naive and misdirected. My preconceived ideas about shifting power and making change in societies were largely political, not personal. I began listening and observing to see how participants were using the capabilities they had developed through the program to make changes in their lives.

One statement in particular, from a female participant, drove home to me the importance of the human element in societal change: 'For once in my life, I was brave enough to tell my de facto of 24 years, I am no longer afraid of him and this is how I am feeling and you have hurt me many times and there is no more doing things your way because you have now got a new Strong Black Woman who is not going to take s#!& anymore'. She explained her transformation by telling her partner that he 'must blame Family Wellbeing because they have shown me a most positive approach'. The penny dropped. I realised that it is, in fact, highly political to teach people the personal skills, knowledge and attitudes necessary to ensure that their human needs were adequately met in life and that they are strong enough to improve their situation. The phrase, 'the personal is political', first used in relation to feminism and Black feminism, was very relevant in Indigenous communities too. Without personal agency, there can be no political or social change. The FWB program in Alice Springs was delivered to health workers and providers of welfare, youth and other services. The intention was to support this group of people—the 'helpers'—to improve their own social and emotional health, thereby enhancing their capacity to support others. It was envisioned that they could become role models, showing young people and their families how to improve their own wellbeing.

The learning approach of FWB relies on the metaphor of life as a physical journey or a form of travel. Starting a new stage in life or work is like embarking on a journey. One needs to plan carefully, think about the destination and how, why and when one will get there. The traveller needs to plan how far they can go and what resources they will need. When travelling with other people, there must be clarity about who is doing what and the options and consequences if someone fails to play their expected role. An important message in the program is that whatever one sets out to do in life, the starting point should always be the establishment of ground rules to determine what is possible or important, and what is not; what is appropriate and what is not; and what is desirable and what is not. Finally, when the journey ends, travellers reflect on and remember experiences and lessons learnt, considering how they may do things better in the future. Essentially, people must understand the parameters of their journey and their own capabilities to be able to travel safely, comfortably and enjoyably from A to B.

The idea that people must be aware of personal strengths and be able to meet their own needs to enable them to help others is a principle that applies equally to those conducting research as it does to those being researched. The aim of FWB is to foster communication, self-reflection and analytic skills to empower people to create support networks, develop resilience and resolve apparently insurmountable problems using creativity and innovation. This aim could be applied to almost any social research project. The FWB program uses the tool of questioning extensively and involves journal writing, pair sharing and group discussion. These methods are used to introduce, develop and reflect on ideas. The FWB journey has several stops along the way before the destination—final stage—is reached. These stops are:

- Formation of a group agreement.
- Identification of human qualities and consideration of how they are used.
- Examination of basic human needs.
- Recounting an individual's life journey.
- Awareness of beliefs and attitudes.
- Grief, loss and conflict resolution.
- Realising the complexity and interconnectedness of human relationships.

After the destination is reached, follow-up and support are provided at regular intervals for program participants to recall and reflect on the journey.

Since my first exposure to FWB, I have taken the journey myself many times, and it has helped me to build projects and drive change. My first journey is my most memorable. The process helped me to find a way to continue to support the aspirations of my home community in Ghana even though I had moved to Australia. It also, as I explain here, eased some financial and personal frustrations. As an academic in Australia in the 1990s, there was much pressure on me to help family and friends back in Ghana who were in financial need. That pressure remains today. Everybody thought I had money; so the demands were endless, and the more I sent money, the more I became frustrated. During an FWB conflict resolution session, I drew on the ground rules and basic human needs topics to help resolve the turmoil I was experiencing. In the first stage of FWB, a group agreement is formed. Workshop sessions involve sharing personal opinions and stories. So the first step is to create an environment where people of diverse backgrounds and belief systems are confident that all points of view will be treated with respect and that people can agree to disagree. Participants therefore negotiate group agreements that define ground rules and set boundaries for what is and what is not acceptable.

In the next step, basic human qualities are identified. Participants consider people they know—friends and family—and identify the qualities they admire in others. Recognising that personal qualities and capabilities are the most important resources one has to work with, participants reflect on the human qualities that each person involved in the journey can contribute. The remarkable thing is that no matter the context in which this exercise is done—whether among women, men and children; parenting groups, workers and managers in Aboriginal organisations; university students in Australia, Papua New Guinea or China; or senior health managers and executives in Timor-Leste—the same qualities are valued. We admire people because they are kind, open, hardworking, enthusiastic, passionate, fair, forgiving, ambitious, clever, wise, humble, brave, modest, empathic and non-judgemental. We admire people who make things better for others. We do not like or admire people who are selfish, or think only of themselves. We do not admire bullies or abusive or aggressive people or those who are quarrelsome, moody, depressive and emotionally demanding. The people we admire are not perfect. They have their flaws, including some of the qualities we do not like. Yet they also have qualities that we admire. These valued qualities are universal and transcend national, ethnic, gender, class, religious and other cultural boundaries.

For me, as I considered my own situation with family and friends back in Ghana, a turning point came when I decided that, like any other initiative in life, I needed to set my own ground rules. I wanted to be a person who helps others, but I needed to guide how I supported others and, where possible, make these rules known to the people who were asking for assistance. Being one of the first to access higher education in my extended family created huge income gaps between myself and others. In my community there was a cultural expectation that whatever belonged to one person in the family belonged to the whole family. I accepted the ethical and cultural responsibility of this expectation from an early age. I understood it was desirable and even noble to use a proportion of my income for the benefit of others, whether family or not. In considering my own situation and how best I could use and apply my human strengths and qualities while maintaining my basic needs, I decided, quite simply and logically, that 'needs' rather than 'wants' would, as much as possible, guide my own patterns of consumption in life. There is a distinct difference between what we want and actually need, materially or otherwise, to live fulfilled and flourishing lives. As humans, however, our wants are unlimited and insatiable. Having taken these foundational steps and decisions, I was confronted with an even bigger dilemma. What was the most ethical way of rationing the relatively limited resources at my disposal in relation to the ever-increasing, and often urgent, needs surrounding me? No matter how hefty the salary packet, I was still only one individual in the midst of countless people in desperate need. It was simply not possible for me to meet everyone's needs.

The remainder of the FWB course expands on how to develop, nurture and apply these human qualities to work and life and routinely assess whether or not they are making a difference. To do this, participants are invited to develop a close awareness of the basic human needs required to live fulfilled lives: physical, emotional, mental and spiritual (Table 5.1). Two things become clear quickly. The more our basic needs are met, the greater our capacity to express our human qualities. The less our basic needs are met, the more our positive qualities are suppressed, leading to our thoughts, actions and relationships becoming increasingly characterised by negative emotions, fear, conflict and addiction.

Following on from these discussions of general universal truths about basic human needs, the focus moves to the personal in FWB. Participants consider their individual life journeys. Using a timeline, they look at their life histories as far back as they can remember and critically reflect on key turning points, in particular the opportunities and adversity they have faced and how they have managed these circumstances. By this time, participants are often ready to start thinking about changes that they would like to make, and they begin examining their own beliefs and attitudes. Do they help us or hinder us from moving on in life? Participants ask where these personal beliefs and attitudes have come from, how reliable these

Table 5.1 Areas of basic human need

Physical: Food, water, shelter, clothing, cleanliness, physical safety, touch and sexual expression
Emotional: To be accepted, understood, supported, valued, respected and recognised; to have self-esteem, confidence and self-worth; to freely express anger, sadness and fear; to give from the heart and take without guilt; to love ourselves and others and build trusting relationships
Mental: To speak freely, think independently, question information, show curiosity; to have choices, to agree or disagree without restriction; to have opinions valued; to continue learning throughout life; to be allowed to make mistakes; to be able to be silent; and to be able to change our minds on an issue or decision
Spiritual: To be deeply connected with our inner self; to be deeply connected with others; to have meaning and purpose in life; to be able to grow, change and express who we truly are; to have in our lives beauty, harmony, generosity, balance, order, truth, creativity, justice, unconditional love, joy, freedom and peace

sources are, whether these beliefs have changed over time and, if so, how. More often than not, these topics lead to acknowledgement and questioning of experiences of loss, grief and resolution of conflicts.

An important part of the FWB process, particularly in Indigenous communities, is learning about and managing responses to trauma—those intense personal responses to loss, death and grief that are a defining feature of a human being's beliefs and attitudes. Grief, loss and conflict resolution are important elements of trauma-informed practice. Understanding how loss affects an individual and understanding how to express grief helps people to heal from trauma, and face relationships and conflicts with courage and openness. Grief and loss are not associated exclusively with traumatic events or deaths of loved ones. Grief and loss can be triggered by the breakdown of a relationship, even a cruel put-down. Human relationships come next. Activities in this part of the program remind everybody that, as humans, relationships enable and limit one's capabilities. These relationships are never confined to two entities. For every relationship between two people or parties, there is at least one more person or entity whose actions and behaviours affect the nature and quality of the relationship.

Having gone through all of the foundation steps of FWB myself, I was ready to address my own dilemmas. I decided the best way to help people in my home village in Ghana and elsewhere was to help them to help themselves. I would not give money to satisfy immediate consumption needs no matter how essential (with the exception of the frail, aged and disabled). A key element of the ground rules I was setting was based on a saying of the Ewe people from my home village in Ghana: 'A person must be willing to lift their own load to knee level before others could help lift it from there onto the head'. In other words, in a situation where needs are huge and the available resources limited, I could not afford to help everyone in need to start doing something from the very beginning. I chose to value-add to people's established efforts instead of helping them to start new things. For example, if a person managed to send their child to school or to begin apprenticeship training for a trade, and halfway through, the going became too difficult through no fault of theirs, I was happy to come to their aid. But if a child needed to start school or learn a trade, I would only come to the party if other family members could get together and meet me halfway. If a person was already trading, then I was happy to assist them to expand or diversify. The idea here was to focus on people who showed potential with the hope that they too would be able to support at least themselves and possibly others. Hence, I treated any support I gave to people as an investment with the expectation that it would yield returns. I did not define these returns narrowly in terms of profit, but rather I defined return as something that enhanced the capacity of the beneficiary to become more self-reliant. The ethics of the right and wrong of supporting only those who show potential can be debated ad nauseam. For me, however, such boundaries gave me clarity about what was possible and what was not. It also helped me to maintain my own sanity. It became clear to me through the sharing process that the Indigenous workers participating in the FWB were experiencing similar cultural pressures as I was from their extended families because of their work and wages. While having an income is good for health and wellbeing, income disparities, combined with cultural expectations, can be stressful, requiring explicit ground rules as to what is possible and what is not.

The remainder of the FWB course focuses on encouraging, supporting and challenging participants to use the foundational knowledge gained to accept and manage change and to better understand and manage challenges and opportunities. Participants are introduced to a range of resources to help plan and monitor changes in their lives, such as mindfulness, visualisation techniques, guides to resolving conflict and priority-setting tools. For example, to prioritise activities, participants may make four lists: things to *start* doing, *stop* doing, do *more* and do *less*. To bring the course to an end, participants are reminded of the core FWB principles, and, depending on resources and logistics, participants are followed up at 6, 12, 18 and 24 months.

I myself went on to establish a Botoku Educational Trust designed to improve access to and quality of education. I used the same ground rules I had come up with during my FWB journey. I invested a set amount per year, and, if the trust managers raised their own funds, I would match this. The Trust has, over the years, invested in chairs, canopies and mattresses, which they hire out at events such as festivals and funerals throughout the district, and it works with extended families to support needy students on the condition that families themselves mobilise to put something on the table. The Trust has been in place since 2000 and is the key education advocate for my home village, Botuku, a highlight of their work being the establishment of a technical/vocational senior high school from 2016.

Bibliography

Aboriginal Education Development Branch. (2002). *Family Wellbeing curriculum document, stages 1–5.* Adelaide: Department of Education, Training and Development.

Tsey, K. (2000). An innovative family support program by and for indigenous Australians: Reflections in evaluation practice. *Journal of Family Studies, 6*(2), 302–308. https://doi.org/10.5172/13229400.2000.11003842.

Tsey, K., & Every, A. (2000). Evaluating Aboriginal empowerment programs – the case of Family Wellbeing. *Australian and New Zealand Journal of Public Health, 24,* 509–514. https://doi.org/10.1111/j.1467-842X.2000.tb00501.x.

Whiteside, M., Bould, E., Tsey, K., Venville, A., Cadet-James, Y., & Morris, M. E. (2017). Promoting twenty-first-century student competencies: A wellbeing approach. *Australian Social Work, 70*(3), 324–336. https://doi.org/10.1080/0312407X.2016.1263351.

Facilitating Empowerment: The Family Wellbeing Program in Alice Springs

Abstract

There are no easy strategies to manage complex challenges (so-called wicked problems) such as colonial dispossession of Indigenous people of their lands and the associated prejudice, discrimination, poverty, trauma and loss. As a researcher working in environments such as these, you must understand the importance of trauma-informed approaches in enabling people not only to heal from past hurt and pain but also to be able to live flourishing lives. Trauma-informed interventions such as the Family Wellbeing program address the psychosocial dimensions of trauma. They take a strengths-based approach whereby people regain a sense of empowerment and control over their lives. In this story, I describe my early efforts to measure the extent and degree of change possible with personal empowerment programs using social research in Alice Springs. I learned many lessons, often through frustration, about the nature of personal empowerment and the ways in which empowerment programs and research might be used more effectively to generate wider-reaching structural and political change in communities.

No matter how desperate a situation may look to the outsider, there are always pockets of strength to be found where people are striving to make things better not only for themselves but also for those around them. Researchers need to seek out and engage such centres of strength because people gain confidence as they become aware of their own strengths. Once people see these strengths and recognise them as resources, they can begin to see a way to tackle hitherto intractable problems. I evaluated an empowerment program deployed in Alice Springs—the Family Wellbeing program (FWB; described in Chap. 5)—in response to high rates of suicide among young men. My goal in the evaluation process was to identify and describe the pockets of strength in the community that had been brought out through the FWB program. Evaluating this program was an interesting and frustrating

© Springer Nature Switzerland AG 2019
K. Tsey, *Working on Wicked Problems*,
https://doi.org/10.1007/978-3-030-22325-0_6

challenge. The budget necessitated a creative approach. I struggled to contextualise the fragmented, stop-start conditions under which the program team was working. In my work at the Menzies School of Health Research, I had used research methods to evaluate a range of health, education and community projects. Those evaluations, which involved devising a tailored measurement and procedural approach and assessing and analysing the effectiveness of the program, were typically funded in the range of $20,000–150,000. Total funding for evaluation of FWB—the first Aboriginal-designed program I had evaluated—was a meagre $3000.

Also challenging was the nature of the FWB intervention. How would I gauge and quantify the benefits, impact and effects of a program that was using individual empowerment to drive societal change? And why were the timeframes and resources devoted to this task so limited and inconsistent? These were very big questions, and my budget was very small. I asked participants for their advice about the best way to capture their experience of the FWB program. I asked: 'I hear all of the benefits you are describing, but what is the best way of finding out and describing the effect of FWB on your life?' They said that, for Aboriginal people, it was important to consider a person within their relationships to others; so we should examine the impact of their participation in FWB on their family and community. They said also that story-telling was important for Aboriginal people and suggested that we consider having them tell their experiences in story form.

On my earliest readings of the materials, it was quite clear that this program had real potential to improve health and wellbeing. Each week, the 31 participants (most of whom were women) reported back to the class on the ways they were using their newly acquired capabilities to deal with parenting issues and relationships with their partners and other extended family members, in their workplaces and in the broader community. By way of example, one woman said, 'Within weeks after starting this course, I had to divorce my family. I'm not talking about my husband; I'm talking about my extended family. Now I can set ground rules. I say to them, it doesn't matter if you are my brother or cousin; if you are drunk you cannot come to my house to demand food. If you are sober you can come. But if you are drunk, it is not fair on my children. This is my ground rule. If you want to maintain a relationship with me, then you have to respect it … It was hard to keep saying no to family. It breaks my heart. Now they accept it and they give me and my children respect.'

To manage within the evaluation budget of $3000, we agreed that every individual would keep a diary (all participants said they could read and write) in which they would describe, using real-life situations, the different ways they had used the FWB ideas and skills within the family, in the workplace or in the wider community. I encouraged them to pose and answer questions through their stories. For example, they might explain how they used an idea or skill, what happened, what the response was, what they did next, what worked well and not so well and things that they would do differently in the future. I said there would also be focus group discussions towards the end of the course. I supplemented this information with a literature review of youth suicide prevention to try to gauge the extent to which the FWB attributes and learning competencies resonated with such programs. Together, these data would form the basis of the program evaluation.

What emerged from the overall analysis of the FWB participants' feedback is that participants had started using their enhanced personal empowerment to tackle relationships and challenges in their lives in ways they previously regarded as impossible for them. Typical comments included: 'Family Wellbeing approach is good because it does not give information from your history to overwhelm you … it makes you see the strengths for the future'; and this one: 'I considered myself illiterate. I was pretty insecure. Once I did FWB I had more than I believed I had. Then I went to college and studied counselling. I had to write assignments. I hadn't been to school since I was 14'; and a third perspective, 'It's helped me with my kids. Realising that they're people and they have feelings and needs too. They need to be listened to too. Before I was stressed out with home life and family—them turning up wanting food and money. Now I put things aside and forget about my worries and give them more time. I'm starting to find out what their needs are because I've slowed down'. Greater confidence to negotiate family relationships was one theme that emerged in the narratives.

The course also had a profound effect on people's relationships and their confidence to deal with workplace issues. In some cases, participants left unsupportive work environments to become self-employed. One participant resigned from her job because she had realised through doing the FWB course that she couldn't work in a non-supportive structure. The effects on her emotional health were too great. She later proudly explained that by doing the course, she had come to appreciate her strengths and expertise and was working for different agencies on a consultancy basis. This was something that, as an Aboriginal woman, she would not have considered before doing the course. Her ultimate aim was to become a full-time teacher in the FWB program 'because of the empowerment it gives people'. Another person had used the skills to deal with workplace conflicts. She was a victim of a serious physical threat and had been accused of being racist, an accusation that caused her deep mental hurt. She wrote: 'Due to the Family Wellbeing course, I feel that I have healed considerably, although in writing up these two incidents I have found many emotions to come back and haunt me. My working life has improved immensely due to a lot of effort put into it by me personally … What I actually love most of all is that I feel so free, alive, energetic, focused, and of being so aware of the many things around me'.

While structural barriers such as institutional racism and poverty still existed, the overwhelming response among participants was that although they might not be able to bring about wide changes in society, they could see how change had begun to take place within themselves and those around them. They felt optimistic that the process would spread. Pockets of strength and inspiration were spawning new ideas and new hope. In Alice Springs, the changes and transformations occurring in participants were also noticed by people close to them, as described by family members and friends: 'She became a lot more active in local Aboriginal politics. She became more involved in her family's struggle for Native Title. She became more confident because she understood it more' (man commenting on partner); 'She thinks more now. She sits down and thinks. If there's a problem, there are steps to follow, there's a right way to do things. She's much more educated to do that' (mother commenting on daughter); and 'She's now developed skills that she's aware that she's able to assist and guide people in making decisions, identifying what their needs are and taking steps. She's just a beautiful person' (friend commenting on a participant).

I began to wonder about the greater potential of the program, particularly if it was conducted with a whole-of-organisation or whole-of-community approach. I was not the only one to whom this idea had occurred. People from Aboriginal Australian communities attending FWB workshops suggested in their course evaluation feedback that FWB would be a useful experience for community leaders, such as local councillors and directors or managers of Aboriginal organisations. Importantly, they also believed that it would equip and prepare non-Indigenous Australians, especially those working with Indigenous people in education, welfare, housing, law, health and employment training, to work more effectively with Indigenous people and to facilitate mutual understanding and reconciliation between Indigenous and other Australians.

The change in people that was being expressed through the evaluation process gave me pause. In my mind, these stories of empowerment fed into a much bigger conversation about 'soft skills' and the pace of change in the world. At the time, I was hearing and reading about twenty-first-century skills, sustainability skills or, perhaps more accurately, emotional intelligence quotient (EQ). These conversations were being had in academic institutions, workplaces and schools all around the world. Societies, communities, economies, environment and culture were changing so rapidly educators and researchers had identified that new skills were needed in this new world. The etiquette of life, the rules, were changing dramatically in so many different sectors of community, and it appeared that people and professions were not keeping up as effectively and as well as they needed to. The ability to learn, change and innovate creatively was being discussed as potentially being far more important than 'hard skills' that might become outdated before a university degree was even completed. The soft skillset reflects a mindset that allows people to be creative and to use innovation and enterprise or leadership to adapt to and/or drive change. Experts were divided, however, about whether or not these skills could be taught. What I was seeing, however, in evaluating this program, was that people were developing a capacity to problem-solve and adapt to change. They were taking relatively simple steps through the program that were allowing them to navigate very complex situations in their personal lives. They were learning soft skills and using them to create happier, more productive homes and relationships.

The individual changes I noticed in Alice Springs, though heartening and positive, were also leading to frustration. The sparks of hope generated in people were beginning to go out soon after they were lit: 'The start-stop-start is frustrating ... each time funding runs out we have to wait for more funding. Why can't we get continuing funding? This is people's lives we are talking about.' Individuals were making changes in themselves but were frustrated by the lack of momentum to translate these personal changes into something more. As one person put it: 'With a lot of our problems amongst the Aboriginal community, we as a people have to come together ... not just as people but as organisations. We need to be working more closely for the betterment of people. Through that FWB, all other services can be used in a better way. Then that healing can take place. Organisations need to come together then families can get on. I know that people are healing through FWB. It is making changes to individuals, but I'm looking bigger. It needs to come from somewhere else as well'.

The idea that bigger changes needed to come from somewhere else highlighted to me the complex nature of empowerment. What I was seeing was that development of soft skills and new capabilities was not simply a means to navigate one's life more effectively; it could also be an agent of societal change. If people could learn these capabilities, and use them to make changes in their immediate environments, what might be achieved if this flexibility, creativity, innovation and confidence could be employed more widely? Empowerment was improving situations for individuals, families and single issues, but was not leading to longer-term structural or societal change in Alice Springs. The personal was not becoming political. In Alice Springs, there was a need for follow-up community mobilisation and development approaches that engaged and enabled participants to use their newfound empowerment to work collaboratively with community leaders to build healthier communities. As a researcher, I could see that, in order to strengthen the research evidence, we needed to take a longer-term approach, well beyond the one-off Alice Springs project funding. It was this long-term approach and planning that was missing in Alice Springs. Delivery and evaluation of the program was largely sporadic and dependent on the availability of short-term funding. Moreover, there was no opportunity to track and assess the longer-term contribution of FWB to improving the protective factors and minimising the risk factors for suicide.

Chapters 7 and 8 examine the challenges and opportunities involved in efforts to apply a longer-term, two-step whole-of-community approach to empowerment. This entailed training a social health workforce using FWB learning modules within a fledgling community-controlled health service, involving the managers through to the health workers. This was followed by the facilitation of community development and Participatory Action Research processes designed to support management and staff to utilise their newfound empowerment and motivation to come together and collectively address issues of high-priority concern to their community.

Bibliography

Every, A., Williams, E., & Tsey, K. (2002). *'Caring and sharing, arntearntearemeleantheme': Family Wellbeing community report.* Alice Springs: University of Queensland School of Population Health, Cairns &Tangentyere Council.

Tsey, K. (2000). An innovative family support program by and for Indigenous Australians: reflections in evaluation practice. *Journal of Family Studies, 6*(2), 302–308. https://doi.org/10.5172/13229400.2000.11003842.

Tsey, K., & Every, A. (2000a). Evaluating Aboriginal empowerment programs – the case of Family Wellbeing. *Australian and New Zealand Journal of Public Health, 24,* 509–514. https://doi.org/10.1111/j.1467-842X.2000.tb00501.x.

Tsey, K., & Every, A. (2000b). Evaluation of an Aboriginal empowerment program. In *Cooperative research centre for Aboriginal and tropical health occasional papers series, 1*. Darwin: Cooperative Research Centre for Aboriginal and Tropical Health.

Tsey, K., & Every, A. (2000c). *Taking control: A summary report for Family Wellbeing graduates*. Darwin & Alice Springs: Cooperative Research Centre for Aboriginal and Tropical Health and Tangentyere Council.

Building Readiness for Change: The Case of Yarrabah Men's Group

7

Abstract

There is no perfect time to engage communities of people in research. Serendipity is at the core of research engagement. Some of the most fulfilling projects or innovative solutions on which I have worked come from serendipitous situations: seeing possibilities and having the will and courage to take a risk and follow them up. As well as intellect, one must use intuition and gut feeling to seize opportunities and make the most of them. Communities and organisations may be interested in working with researchers, but it is not always obvious to them exactly how research may serve their needs and aspirations. The key is to create relationships that are based on deep listening, empathy and honesty. Ask what potential partners are doing and how research may add value. Researchers must put themselves in their partners' shoes and imagine the challenges and opportunities they are facing. Through this understanding, researchers and research communities can envisage how research may strengthen what is being done. This story explains how a chance encounter with Yarrabah Men's Group leaders laid the foundation for enduring research partnerships with significant social health benefits for a whole community.

The year was 2000. The place was Cairns. I was 1 week into a new job. I was meeting many different people. A colleague, Ernest Hunter, introduced me to a man called Les Baird, a Minister in his church, manager of a fledgling community-controlled health service and one of a handful of community leaders supporting a local men's group. Les was from Yarrabah, a beach town about 50 km south of the city of Cairns in Far North Queensland. Les was quick to see an opportunity, and soon after our introductions, he asked me: 'When are you coming to Yarrabah to give a talk to our Men's Group?'. He said the group met every 2 weeks on Wednesday evenings at 7 pm for 1 or 2 h. 'Give me your phone number and I'll arrange for you to come and talk to us.'

© Springer Nature Switzerland AG 2019   41
K. Tsey, *Working on Wicked Problems*,
https://doi.org/10.1007/978-3-030-22325-0_7

I had never heard of men's groups before so I had a lot of questions. Firstly, what was a men's group? What sort of men belongs to the group? What should I talk about? Is this a backlash against the women's movement? How many people are likely to be there? What about my accent? Will they understand me and will I understand them? Will I need an interpreter? All of these questions were going through my mind, but my new friend didn't seem particularly worried. He continued reiterating: 'Just come ... you can talk about anything. Some of the previous guest speakers did presentations on the importance of good nutrition, physical activity, safe sex, alcohol, smoking and suicide prevention. The men enjoyed learning about all these things, so don't you worry. Just come and talk about anything you wish. You can even talk about Africa'.

I am somebody who likes to think things through carefully before acting, and it was not at all clear to me what I was committing myself to. Nevertheless, I said, 'Sure, I'd love to come to Yarrabah and give a talk. This is my number; please give me a call so we can arrange a date.' A week later I got a call from Les. He said he had told the men about me and that I should come the following Wednesday at about 6 pm for a barbecue before the talk. He gave me directions to get to Yarrabah, and I said I was looking forward to the visit. The idea of visiting a beautiful place and meeting new people was, of course, appealing but I was anxious, and I still had no idea what to talk about.

I turned to my colleagues, who had worked in Yarrabah and other similar Aboriginal communities, for guidance. They advised me to select one of my previous research projects and to use visual props such as photographs and graphs to make the presentation interesting. I chose a favourite topic of mine at the time: the link between schooling and health outcomes. This research was conducted mainly in developing countries in the 1970s and 1980s; it showed that the level of education of the parents largely determined the health outcomes of their children. The relationship was very strong in the case of mothers and their children and also, to some degree, fathers. I was interested in people's views and whether they thought the relationships might be the same in Aboriginal communities.

The Wednesday came and after finishing work at 5 pm, I set off for Yarrabah. Before I knew it, I had driven past the turnoff and found myself off-track. Luckily, a local person was kind enough to redirect me via a shortcut, so I was not too late. There were around ten people at the barbecue when I arrived and I thought, 'Good, I can handle this number'. But then, in twos and threes, more people began to appear. After the barbecue I found myself sitting in front of about 30 men in a classroom situation, being introduced by my new friend, who said that I was going to talk about education and health. Of course, all the men were now waiting eagerly for me to start performing. At that point I said to myself: 'Quick, I have to do something.' Firstly, I said: 'Please, is it OK if we rearrange the chairs so we can all sit in one large circle, instead of me being up here in front of you like a teacher?' Then I said: 'Starting with Les, who has just introduced me, please let's go around the circle so that everybody has the opportunity, if they wish, to explain who they are. Could you share with me some of the Men's Group activities you have been involved in, and some of the things that you are hoping the group will achieve in the future?'

By the time it came to my turn, I had learned so much, not only about the group, but also about the broader community. I learned a sad story of their community: from the 1980s Yarrabah had been confronted with waves of suicide. Similar to the situation in Alice Springs, discussed in Chaps. 5 and 6, it was mainly young men who were taking their lives, in what was called copy-cat fashion. As soon as one person attempted or committed suicide, others followed. Most local people felt that this tragedy was a new development in the history of the community. People were frustrated that any time Yarrabah appeared in the news, it was about the fact that the community had one of the highest suicide rates in the world. Yet there had been very few organised efforts to deal with the problem. In the absence of outside help, a group of local people had mobilised themselves, saying 'Enough is enough'. The community closed down the alcohol canteen and, with the support of mental health professionals, set up a crisis response team of 'life promotion officers'. The community planned to set up its own health service so people would have access to the social and emotional wellbeing services seen as important at that time.

It was from this situation of suicide and sadness that the Men's Support Group had grown. About half a dozen men had suggested they should come together to try to provide positive role models for younger people. They wanted to give them hope, to empower them to be comfortable with their Aboriginal identity and to teach them to be strong and resilient. By the time I first visited the Men's Group, they had been meeting fortnightly for nearly 2 years. There were between 7 and 12 men who attended regularly and many more who attended when there was a guest speaker. Yarrabah's vision was to have its own community-controlled health service. A health feasibility study had identified 'loss of spirit' as a major cause of suicide in the community and recommended a 'social, emotional, and spiritual health centre of excellence' as key to efforts to prevent suicide. Les Baird was the manager of this health service, the Gurriny Yealamucka Health Service (Gurriny), which was established in name only at that stage. It was his job to work with the Yarrabah Council to implement the community-controlled health idea. The people of Yarrabah believed that a community-controlled health service was important to address social health issues such as the suicide epidemic, but they were not confident in their capacity to run a full medical health service.

I thanked the men for sharing so much with me in such a short time and said that it had allowed me to gain a better understanding of their group. I told them a little more about myself that I was from Ghana, how long I had been in Australia, the places I had lived and a few of the research projects in which I had been involved, including the Alice Springs Family Wellbeing (FWB) evaluation. From listening to their stories, I could see the men shared the same pain and problems that I had witnessed in Alice Springs. I thought they might be interested in experiencing for themselves a piece of the program that was being used in Alice Springs. This diversion went against my usual modus operandi of detailed planning in advance, but I sensed an opportunity and knew I had an interested and attentive audience. I said: 'Instead of giving you the talk I had prepared, how about I give you a small taste of the Family Wellbeing program?' When they agreed I gave the group two simple mental exercises, one relating to the FWB 'Human Qualities' topic and one to 'Basic Human Needs'.

I asked them first of all to think about their families. 'You can define family any way you like: parents, siblings, children, grandparents, cousins, uncles, nieces, nephews and close friends who feel like family. Among all the people in your family, think carefully about one person that you really admire and respect. Then think about the types of things or qualities you admire and respect most about that person.' I gave them some time. 'Secondly, think about your work or other settings like church or your Men's Group and, again, identify a person you respect. Think about the things that you admire about them.' There was a third piece of the activity: 'Finally, think about yourself – what are some of the things that you admire and respect about yourself?' I asked them to take a few minutes to reflect quietly on the three tasks and then to turn to the person next to them and share whatever information they felt comfortable talking about. I asked them to take turns to talk to each other for up to 5 min, and then we shared thoughts in the larger group. Through the exercise, participants discovered that the people they admired universally were kind, open-minded or hardworking; they did not give up easily. Some had achieved recognition in life, while others were quiet achievers in the sense that they simply got on with what they needed to do without fuss and attention, yet they all demonstrated some admirable qualities.

For the topic covering basic human needs, I asked them to think about the four types of basic human needs: physical, emotional, mental and spiritual. I said that physical needs included things like food, exercise, shelter, sexual expression and adequate sleep. Emotional needs included feeling safe, giving and receiving respect and love and feeling valued and appreciated. Mental needs included curiosity about the world and the opportunity to learn throughout life. On a spiritual level, people needed to be connected to something bigger than themselves. Ideally, I explained, we should be able to enjoy a life of beauty, creativity, peace and tranquillity. I then asked them to identify some of the basic human needs that they thought were being met in their lives and describe how this made them feel. I also asked them to consider needs that were not being met so well and describe how this made them feel. Finally, I asked what steps they themselves could take to ensure their basic human needs were met better.

I then explained that from the FWB's point of view, the more they understood about the importance of meeting basic human needs, the more they would see the qualities that they admired in themselves and others flourish. I reminded them to view their human qualities as very special resources that were freely available for them to cultivate and use. They were pleasantly surprised when I said that they did not need money to acquire these qualities and that although money might help to nurture their development, it was not essential. Finally, I explained that the human qualities and basic human needs topics formed the foundation of the FWB, while the rest of the program was about using the foundation knowledge to deal with day-to-day challenges in their lives such as relationships, conflict, emotions, crisis, beliefs and attitudes, loss and grief, addictions, violence and abuse. By then it was almost 10 pm. So I thanked the group for their trust in sharing so much with me.

They thanked me and I drove off into the night, dodging a couple of long snakes on the way.

A week later, Les came back to me. The men were very keen to participate in the full FWB program. 'How much would it cost? Can you work with us to find money and introduce the course to Yarrabah?' he asked. 'Yes, I'd love to do that, but I think there's a lot more we can do together. Your community is trying to do something important, and the world needs to know how much you are achieving, what is standing in the way, and what sort of support you need to achieve your goals. You need to share this information for your own community and for other communities wanting to improve things for themselves so that they can learn from your experience'. I explained to Les that the program would be much more worthwhile, and have further-reaching potential, if it was conducted as a community-driven research project aligned to their community needs. My evaluation of the Alice Springs FWB project, and its potential to be so much more than personal development, was still in my mind. I saw an opportunity in Yarrabah to take a longer-term approach, to make the personal political.

One unanswered question had stuck in my mind after my visit to the Men's Group. I asked Les, 'Before we go on, please tell me why you said the other day at the meeting that the community did not believe in its own ability to run a health service?' He explained that Queensland Health already ran a small hospital that provided clinical services for the community and some people were scared of losing it without anything to replace it. He said the hospital staff dealt in medical matters but showed little understanding of social, emotional and spiritual health. After a lengthy discussion, we agreed that the new Gurriny Health Service and my university research team would work together to develop a Gurriny social, emotional and spiritual health program (social health) to complement Queensland Health's current medical services. We hypothesised that once Gurriny had developed a social health capability, supported by research evidence, Gurriny and the community would have the credibility and confidence in their ability to control their own comprehensive health service.

I explained that the FWB program founders recognised that there were no easy strategies to manage complex challenges such as cross-generational suffering and associated suicide. FWB takes a strength-based approach whereby people regain a sense of empowerment and control over their lives. This helps people to develop a win-win rather than a win-lose mindset, which, in turn, strengthens their capacity to rebuild trust and confidence that may have been damaged by loss and hurt associated with previous conflict and hurt. I said we could use FWB first to help people to heal and better address their day-to-day challenges. Then we could use Participatory Action Research (PAR) to bring FWB participants and other community members together to tackle the issues of greatest concern for the community. PAR is based on the principle that people can become researchers in their own right and generate relevant knowledge to address issues that concern them. I explained to Les that PAR allowed communities of people, supported by researchers, to define and clarify their goals. 'We prioritise those things that your Men's Group and the wider community really want to change. We then plan and take steps to make those changes happen.

Along the way we have to keep reflecting and asking ourselves: What are we trying to do? Why are we doing it? Is there any precedent for what we are trying to do? Who is benefiting from our activities and who is missing out? Is it fair? How do we know if we are achieving our aims?'

Meeting Les was a chance encounter. Having just begun a new job with a heavy teaching load, I was not necessarily looking very hard for new project opportunities. What happened was a serendipitous encounter, recognised and acted upon by both Les and me. We both saw different opportunities from our interaction, and, as life would have it, we both acted upon each of them. The visit to the Yarrabah Men's Group was the catalyst for a long and productive working relationship that has had lasting positive impact on the lives of individuals and of a whole community. My colleagues and I have engaged in FWB and other related research, not only with the men's and women's groups but with virtually the entire Yarrabah community: the health service, the residential alcohol rehabilitation centre, the Yarrabah Council, rangers, youth groups, a dance group and the school. By 2011, some 463 people, 16% of Yarrabah's estimated total population of 3000, had participated in FWB. At the time of writing this book in 2019, the Yarrabah Men's Group and the Gindaja alcohol residential service continue to use FWB as a preventative and rehabilitation program. FWB research contributed, as one of a range of strategies, to a notable reduction in suicide rates in the community.

In Chap. 8 I will explain the contribution of FWB research to suicide reduction in the Yarrabah community. As a result of their successful initiatives, a consortium of FWB researchers and the Yarrabah community received $1.5 million in funding from the National Suicide Prevention Strategy Prime Ministerial Flagship projects, to enable Yarrabah to share its successful suicide prevention experience with other Queensland Indigenous communities.

Bibliography

Mayo, K., Tsey, K., McCalman, J., Whiteside, M., Fagan, R., & Baird, L. (2009). The research dance: University and community research collaborations at Yarrabah, North Queensland, Australia. *Health and Social Care in the Community, 17*, 133–140. https://doi.org/10.1111/j.1365-2524.2008.00805.x.

Prince, J., Jeffrey, N., Baird, L., Kingsburra, S., & Tipiloura, B. (2018). Stories from community: How suicide rates fell in two Indigenous communities. Canberra: Aboriginal & Torres Strait Islander Healing Foundation.

Taking a Long-Term Approach: The Family Wellbeing Program in Yarrabah

8

Abstract

Researchers can become deeply committed to their interventions and to their research communities. This kind of long-term, sustained relationship between researchers and the people with whom they work is useful in communities where historical trauma or entrenched social disadvantage is evident and solutions will not be found quickly. Researchers cannot expect to unravel or alter, in the course of a 6-month or a 3-year grant period, social or health conditions that have been developing for years (or in some cases, centuries). A sustained research relationship can also lead to a degree of trust and flexibility that cannot be achieved in short-term projects. A research project that is less rigid and more open to change is somewhat messier to manage but also likely to be more responsive to changes in needs and communities. My association with the Aboriginal Family Wellbeing program has been a long one, as has my association with the community of Yarrabah. In this chapter, I use examples from my Family Wellbeing work in Yarrabah to demonstrate how a long-term approach has enabled us to achieve a critical mass of targeted groups to help address complex issues, such as transgenerational trauma and the associated issues of drug and alcohol abuse, domestic violence and suicide.

Demonstrating research impact is far more involved than simply reporting research results. It requires a long-term view of program development, delivery and evaluation. My long-standing association with the community of Yarrabah and with my Family Wellbeing (FWB) work has given me a unique lens through which to view the issue of research impact. Throughout the process of considering how to best demonstrate impact, I have reflected on nearly 20 years of involvement in community development research in Yarrabah. Here, I describe the strengths-based, two-step approach we applied in Yarrabah to ensure that the personal empowerment

© Springer Nature Switzerland AG 2019   47
K. Tsey, *Working on Wicked Problems*,
https://doi.org/10.1007/978-3-030-22325-0_8

program being delivered to individuals in the community would translate to greater structural and societal changes, creating a real impact in the community and beyond.

I first helped to bring FWB to the Aboriginal community of Yarrabah, south of Cairns in Far North Queensland, in the early 2000s, following a chance encounter with one of the convenors of a local men's group, as described in Chap. 7. The program has been a feature of community development initiatives in Yarrabah since that time. Different pools of money have been used, different organisations have led programs, various grants have spun off from FWB and people numbering in the hundreds have experienced the program in some form in this relatively small town. In projects in which I was involved, we made a commitment to use half the salary allocation of all research budgets to employ local people as community-based researchers, based on the principle that if research is being done in a given community, then people from the target community should be supported to participate both as researchers and in research governance roles. The downside is a lot of our efforts went into building people's capacity for research, and in a highly competitive funding environment, this can affect overall research outputs such as publications and, in turn, capacity to attract new grants.

The long-term nature of the town's experience working with FWB has enabled me, as a researcher with a keen interest in program evaluation, to consider the ripple effect of a thoroughly human empowerment-based project in some depth. It has also enabled me to examine the concept and the practicalities of research impact in a very tangible way.

The FWB pilot project took place in Yarrabah between May 2002 and December 2003. The program was adapted to the context and needs of the Yarrabah community, which sought to use it to consider a daunting number of issues, ranging from suicide prevention to inadequate housing and domestic violence to building a local social health workforce. We developed a two-step Participatory Action Research (PAR) process, whereby community members became researchers in their own right, as described in Chap. 7. Step 1 involved structured personal development training workshops for key community service providers, leaders and community members, based on the foundation topics of the Aboriginal-developed FWB program. Step 2 involved follow-up community mobilisation and development of processes aimed at supporting groups of FWB participants to lead and collectively address identified high-priority community issues arising out of the personal development training.

A total of 55 people participated in the FWB pilot workshops: 34 men and 21 women. Ten people, five men and five women, went on to complete the facilitator training program. Researchers and the ten newly qualified local facilitators then went on to conduct the FWB program in partnership with a variety of community groups: a women's group, a men's group, a youth group, a school and a drug and alcohol rehabilitation centre. Participants were recruited through word of mouth, posters in public locations and letters to relevant organisations and interested individuals. Each workshop commenced with the development of a group agreement, which committed members to certain guidelines for working together. The workshops operated using a strengths-based approach. The main building blocks of strengths-based practice include a focus on trusting and workable relationships; the empowerment of people to take a lead in their solution finding; working collaboratively on mutually agreed goals; and drawing on the personal/communal resources of motivation and hope and the creation of sustainable change through learning and experiential growth. In a holistic strengths-based approach, research users become coresearchers in their own right, using the experiences and knowledge they are gaining to improve their situation in a meaningful and sustainable way.

In Yarrabah, evaluation research showed that strengths-based approaches were making a difference. In-depth interviews were conducted with the various participant groups 6–12 months after their participation in FWB. Those who were interviewed spoke repeatedly of a newfound insight that they needed to heal and understand their own problems before they could help others. For one participant the course provided the opportunity to explore painful memories of sexual abuse experienced as a child and enabled him to confront these issues so as to deal with them more constructively: 'I'm coming out of healing from sexual abuse. And that is another good thing from that course … it helped me understand about sexual abuse'. Another remarked, 'I had not heard anything about it [referring to the FWB program] before but just going through the contents and that, I got the immediate impression that it is more like a personal healing development program. I think that's what makes it so good because if you're going to help somebody else then you have to get yourself right first, and that [FWB] was a step in the right direction. For me, especially in the area that I work in, Men's Health and supporting men, I just needed to get myself right before I could talk to others and help others'. Step 1 was going to plan.

Step 2 in the research capacity-building process was much bigger and more complicated. Through the FWB workshops, participants identified a range of opportunities and problems that were making life difficult for them, their families and their neighbours. Some of these issues were gravely important at a very basic level; for example, some people did not have safe housing. Projects identified included working with the school to tackle poor attendance rates, developing community child-care programs for children at risk, a Yabba Bimbi Men's Dance Group to engage men in meaningful activity and a housing action group designed to address the chronic housing shortage in the community. Others included youth binge drinking and domestic violence. Various programs led by researchers and newly trained facilitators were implemented with varying degrees of success. We supported local people to participate both as paid researchers and to take on unpaid research governance roles. This gave people the opportunity not only to be exposed to research but importantly to re-engage with learning and employment. The downside of this approach is that, when much effort is redirected and allocated to building people's capacity for research, publication outputs can be affected negatively. In turn, this can have an impact on future bids for grants. Each Yarrabah program evolved in its own way, some gradually, others relatively quickly, some neatly and others very messily. One thing most programs did have in common was a consistent approach in the form of the FWB principles and the two-step methodology. In the latter part of this chapter, I have chosen three stories from Yarrabah to illustrate practical ways FWB researchers used a long-term approach to demonstrate the societal impact of their research.

8.1   Case Study 1: The Evolution of Yarrabah Men's Group: Take a Long-Term View by Starting at the Ending

The Yarrabah Men's Group first formed in response to a very high rate of suicide among young men. The vision of the Men's Group, as described in their promotional flyers, was to 'restore men's rightful role in the community using a holistic healing approach encompassing the spiritual, mental, physical, emotional and social aspects of health'. One of the first things we did at the start of the PAR process was to encourage the men to translate their vision statement into concrete achievable goals. What was a man's rightful role in the community? The men, in small groups, were asked to imagine and describe the behaviour patterns of a Yarrabah man who does play his rightful role in community. The results were carefully collated into a list of 'Do's and Don'ts'. An abridged version of the list is included in Table 8.1.

The Do's and Don'ts list gave the men a clear identity and values to which they aspired. It also provided a set of criteria against which to monitor and evaluate the Men's Group activities over time. By creating this list—picturing their end-goal—and using it as a measurement tool, the men in the group could set and achieve incremental goals for themselves and express their progress numerically. They were building their own capacity to think like researchers, planners and community developers. At the start of the project, participants were asked to rate their individual performances and behaviours against the Do's and Don'ts using a simple scale from 0 to 10, 0 being poor and 10 being excellent, and then to give reasons for their ratings. For many people, the concept of Do's and Don'ts was a new one, and the idea that they could move their ratings up was motivating and achievable. After 2 years of involvement, the majority of the men improved their rating against the Do's and Don'ts by at least 4 or 5 points. The two most frequent reasons the men gave for their improvement were personal development through FWB and a greater sense of responsibility for their families.

Yarrabah Men's Group members felt strongly that their own contributions to preventing suicide in the community were productive and useful. At the personal level, men reported having a greater sense of direction; being more aware of their basic needs and what is important and what is not; being more willing to seek help

Table 8.1 Yarrabah Men's Group Do's and Don'ts

Do	Don't
Be loving kind and compassionate	Argue in front of kids
Be forgiving, respectful and truthful	Be lazy and expect everything like a king
Support families by working and paying bills	Gamble money away
Instil confidence in your family	Be a slave to alcohol, drugs, gambling and pleasures of the self
Have clear goals	Hate or reject people or put them down
Be an example to others	Be macho about certain jobs
Spend time with and read to children	Be violent to others and family
Admit when you are wrong	Be selfish

when needed; sharing more in housework; and spending more time with their children. Some men said they had started to do bedtime reading for their children. At an organisational level, the strengthened Men's Group, which was using research methods to record their progress, now brought in resources to implement a range of high-priority community development initiatives. The group had originally formed with suicide prevention in mind, but mental health projects were not necessarily a high priority. The issues went much deeper and, as such, the diverse projects that evolved to address high suicide rates were focused on fulfilling a range of unmet basic needs rather than simply counselling people (although this was one component). These included funding for a 3-year youth empowerment project; seed funding to work with young people to develop a family violence prevention model; and employment of a business manager and choreographer to train members of a newly formed dance group—Yabba Bimbi Men's Cultural Dance Group. At a community level, in a 9-year period, suicide rates dropped from a high of three to four completed suicides per year in the 1990s to two suicides over the entire 9-year period since 1998, when the Men's Group formed. Injury rates also declined. While it is difficult to say exactly how much Men's Group, FWB and other activities contributed to any of these outcomes, a Men's Group leader explained his perception of the role and contribution of their group: 'I reckon Men's Group plays an important preventative role. Life Promotion attends to the immediate crisis because it is set up to provide crisis response. But Men's Group is for the long process of bringing respect and confidence back to men. To show men that they are not alone and it is OK to seek help. Men's Group is for prevention'.

8.2   Case Study 2: Beware the 'Iceberg Issues': Be Prepared to Revisit and Revise Your Goals

Yarrabah FWB participants identified that the basic need of shelter was not being met in their community. One person vividly articulated the plight of a significant number of people, about 25 families, living in tin shacks, with no mains power or water. They depended on generators to provide electricity and on gravity-fed water supply. The roads were unsealed in many areas. People who attended this meeting decided to form themselves into a Housing Group and agreed on an initial action plan. They researched the options available to residents for obtaining resources to build houses themselves with available local labour. They met with the Yarrabah Council, the Aboriginal and Torres Strait Islander Commission and government departments in order to gain a better understanding of the reasons for the desperate housing situation in the community. They spoke with traditional owners about their views on land claims and on mobilising community support in addressing these issues.

As the Housing Group proceeded with strategy development, it became clear that one of the big factors contributing to the lack of historical and current progress was the issue of land tenure. They discovered that funds had been allocated for new housing, but their local council had had to resort to returning this government funding because of the inability to secure land to build new houses. Issues around land tenure arose from historical tensions between traditional owners and other members of the community who were part of the Stolen Generations and were sent to Yarrabah as part of the assimilation policies of the state government. Land tenure and historical rivalries are not quick-fix issues. Progress was slow, it was difficult to make structural changes within the community, and some participants became frustrated and disillusioned. There was one member of the group who expected more immediate results: 'I would like to see more happening – I don't want to be sitting here talking now and 3 years later you come back and we still talking and nothing happening, it's frustrating … I don't like that. Until people down here got nice roofs over their heads with power and water then I'd be a happy man'. However, the complexities of the issues regarding Native Title and obtaining funding from the government were immense. They required careful negotiations among all parties. What started as a project to house families quickly snowballed into something far more complex. The researchers and the community needed to rethink their goals and revise their plans and timeframes, two things that would not have been possible without taking a long-term view.

Despite the frustrations, some real gains were made over the first few years of the Housing Group activities, and the leaders were pleased with the eventual progress: 'It is making a change because the traditional owners and the council were at a stall for a couple of years with arguments and that, but now they are getting it together, sitting down and negotiating'. The FWB Housing Group identified a number of significant achievements. Firstly, the council formally extended the Yarrabah township boundaries to include the outlying areas where the tin shacks were. The effect of this move was that the council made a commitment to provide infrastructure such as roads, water, electricity and other amenities. Some of these infrastructure activities were still being implemented in 2018. Secondly, members of the housing action group, and men's and women's Groups, saw the need to become directly involved in local government to achieve action. One person was elected to the Yarrabah Council, followed by a second who later became mayor, with housing as his top priority. Those involved in the housing action group were not the usual community leaders or spokespeople, and they had never thought of themselves as such. One of these people was pleasantly surprised that 'We're the talk of the town'. This phrase subsequently became the title of a report into the progress of the FWB groups.

8.3   Case Study 3: Evaluation Planning: The First and Last Step in Any Research Project

For some time, the Yarrabah community had been worried about binge drinking, or 'drinking to get drunk', among young people. The situation appeared to be aggravated by the demise of a so-called 'work for the dole' program, Community Development Employment Projects (CDEP), which had occupied young people for 2 days a week. Since the CDEP had stopped, young people had 7 days a week with nothing much to occupy them. Many people believed this was a major cause of the binge drinking. A consortium of Yarrabah organisations had secured Commonwealth Alcohol Education funding to raise awareness among 12- to 25-year-olds about the dangers of binge drinking at existing community events, including sports competitions and carnivals. The initiative was called 'Beat da Binge'.

While the Commonwealth funded the project, there was, as usual, no provision for evaluation beyond the usual process data: the number of events and the number of people who attended. There were many reviews saying we were very good at describing the nature of the problems within Aboriginal health and suggesting steps to fix problems, but were not at all good at implementing reliable evaluations. At the same time, however, there was no funding provided for evaluation. In reviewing Indigenous health publications, including several by our own team, Rob Sanson-Fisher and colleagues found that 80% were mainly descriptive, including mere opinions of individuals, and that only 20% were program and service evaluations, most of which were of poor design quality. I was very frustrated that the Commonwealth Government was perpetuating stories about 'the sorry state of evidence' in Indigenous health research while doing nothing to fund proper evaluations. This lack of proper evaluation by Commonwealth and other funding bodies, which I had come across too often, made me determined to do whatever I could to evaluate initiatives such as the binge drinking project. I just had to apply a bit of initiative and creativity.

We committed to finding small savings from the overall project budget to put towards evaluation. The researchers agreed to supplement this with in-kind contributions. The evaluation was to take a participatory approach, so that emergent findings could be used to improve the ongoing project quality. For this reason, a small evaluation committee comprising the researchers and project managers was formed to provide overall direction to the evaluation. Firstly, we conducted a rapid literature review focusing on young people and binge drinking. The review unearthed some interesting findings. There were hardly any alcohol evaluations related to projects with rural Indigenous youth. The few evaluations that had been done did not provide reliable baseline data against which to evaluate alcohol and harm reduction initiatives among Indigenous youth. This was not helpful. What we did discover from the literature review was that the most effective and economical way to engage young people with interventions such as the binge drinking project was to place the young people themselves squarely at the centre of the project. Until that point, it was adults, mainly service providers, who were organising the Yarrabah *Beat da Binge* events. Not surprisingly, only a few young people attended them.

These findings were presented to the project stakeholders and triggered two important decisions. Firstly, we would implement a reliable community survey to generate baseline data, and, secondly, we would identify, train and employ interested young people to work on the survey and the project. The before and after survey of 12- to 25-year-olds would determine the level of alcohol intake, preferred types of drinks and the places, times, amounts spent and companions associated with drinking patterns. Importantly, the data would provide a rare opportunity for the community to monitor and evaluate their young people's alcohol use and to develop future alcohol prevention initiatives for young people. Evaluation planning and execution was to be both the first and last step in the project and the driver for change in the future.

The results show that *Beat da Binge* was associated with a statistically significant reduction (10%) in the proportion of survey respondents who reported that they had engaged in an episode of short-term risky drinking; reductions (between 4% and 31%) in the frequency of short-term risky drinking for all beverage types except wine; a $6.25 reduction in mean expenditure on alcohol during short-term risky drinking sessions; and a 7% reduction in the proportion of activities with family or friends that usually include alcohol. There were also statistically significant increases in awareness of binge drinking (28%) and of standard drinks (21%). In addition to alcohol-specific outcomes, there was a statistically significant (8%) increase in the proportion of respondents engaged in training as their main weekday activity, which was partly offset by a 13% reduction in those whose main weekday activity was family care or home-related tasks. Reductions in the proportion of survey respondents who reported binge drinking, along with increases in awareness and involvement in alcohol-free social activities, suggest the community-based intervention was effective.

My research relationship with Yarrabah has continued in one form or another to this day. The same can be said for people who have joined my team over the years. For example, at the time of writing this book, two colleagues, whose PhDs I supervised, are leading a new 5-year National Health and Medical Research Council youth mental health intervention; Yarrabah is one of the three intervention sites. These researchers have worked with my team at two different universities, and now lead their own empowerment interventions at another university. Nurturing and sustaining a consistent research workforce on short-term funding is very difficult. Relationships are important, and it simply does not work to contract different researchers on a short-term basis to work on each new project. Apart from the difficulty of attracting the right person at the right time, it is confusing for communities to deal with a new researcher with each new project.

Developing and implementing interventions in Indigenous communities is often more complicated than researchers like to admit. Times change, institutions can change and funding body priorities can change. In the 12-month period between when a grant is developed and successful applications are announced, community priorities can change significantly. Using funds from existing projects to support continuity of staff pending the availability of new funding is often messy. The people within the research communities, however, are less likely to change. Building local capacity is one of the most important and crucial ways to ensure continuity in social research. It is a key enabler in taking a long-term approach. By earmarking a proportion of research salary budgets to employ local people, we were able to build lasting research capacity and local ownership of the research. If we can combine strong research relationships with strong research capacity within the communities themselves, we can hold an intervention firmly in place despite financial, pragmatic or social uncertainties.

Bibliography

Daly, B., Tsey, K., Whiteside, M., Baird, L., Kingsburra, S., Jackson, K., et al. (2004). *'We're the talk of the town': Facilitating mastery and control in indigenous communities. An evaluation of a Family wellbeing personal and community development project in Yarrabah.* Cairns: University of Queensland School of Population Health, and Yarrabah: Gurriny Yealamucka Health Service Aboriginal Corporation.

Jainullabudeen, T. A., Lively, A., Singleton, M., Shakeshaft, A., Tsey, K., McCalman, et al. (2015). The impact of a community-based risky drinking intervention (Beat da Binge) on indigenous young people. *BMC Public Health, 15*(1), 1–7.

Mayo, K., Tsey, K., McCalman, J., Whiteside, M., Fagan, R., & Baird, L. (2009). The research dance: University and community research collaborations at Yarrabah, North Queensland, Australia. *Health and Social Care in the Community, 17*, 133–140. https://doi. org/10.1111/j.1365-2524.2008.00805.x.

McCalman, J., Baird, B., & Tsey, K. (2007). Indigenous men taking their rightful place – How one Aboriginal community is achieving results. *Aboriginal and Islander Health Worker Journal, 31*, 8–9.

McCalman, J., Tsey, K., Bainbridge, R., Shakeshaft, A., Singleton, M., & Doran, C. (2013). Tailoring a response to youth binge drinking in an Aboriginal Australian community: A grounded theory study. *BMC Public Health, 13*, 1–9. https://doi.org/10.1186/1471-2458-13-726.

McCalman, J., Tsey, K., Reilly, L., Connolly, B., Fagan, R., Earles, W., et al. (2010a). Taking control of health: Gurriny's story of organisational change. *Third Sector Review, 16*, 29–47.

McCalman, J., Tsey, K., Wenitong, M., Wilson, A., McEwan, A., Cadet-James, Y., et al. (2010b). Indigenous men's support groups and social and emotional wellbeing: A meta-synthesis of the evidence. *Australian Journal of Primary Health, 16*, 159–166. https://doi.org/10.1071/ PY09032.

Paul, C. L., Sanson-Fisher, R., Stewart, J., & Anderson, A. E. (2010). Being sorry is not enough: The sorry state of the evidence base for improving the health of indigenous populations. *American Journal of Preventive Medicine, 38*(5), 566–568. https://doi.org/10.1016/j. amepre.2010.02.001.

Prince, J., Jeffrey, N., Baird, L., Kingsburra, S., & Tipiloura, B. (2018). Stories from community: How suicide rates fell in two Indigenous communities. Canberra: Aboriginal & Torres Strait Islander Healing Foundation.

Tsey, K., Patterson, D., Whiteside, M., Baird, L., & Baird, B. (2002). Indigenous men taking their rightful place in society? A preliminary analysis of a participatory action research process with Yarrabah Men's Health Group. *Australian Journal of Rural Health, 10*, 278–284. https://doi. org/10.1046/j.1440-1584.2002.00491.x.

Tsey, K., Patterson, D., Whiteside, M., Baird, L., Baird, B., & Tsey, K. (2003). Indigenous men taking their rightful place in society? A follow up report. *Australian Journal of Rural Health, 11*, 285–286. https://doi.org/10.1111/j.1440-1584.2003.tb00554.x.

Tsey, K., Wenitong, M., McCalman, J., Whiteside, M., Baird, L., Patterson, D., et al. (2004). A participatory action research process with a rural Indigenous men's group: Monitoring and reinforcing change. *Australian Journal of Primary Health, 10*, 130–136. https://doi. org/10.1071/PY04057.

Tsey, K., Whiteside, M., Haswell-Elkins, M., Bainbridge, R., Cadet-James, Y., & Wilson, A. (2009). Empowerment and Indigenous Australian health: A synthesis of findings from Family Wellbeing formative research. *Health and Social Care in the Community, 18*, 169–179. https:// doi.org/10.1111/j.1365-2524.2009.00885.x.

Managing Unanticipated Consequences: Historical Research in Ghana

9

Abstract

Research, by its very nature, can have a degree of trial and error about it. We must acknowledge and represent the error as well as the trial. Research engagement and impact are always evolving. One solution can often become a trigger for new challenges. In my research career, I have approached engagement as a life-long activity in much the same way that anthropologists and linguists do, by building relationships with a community over an entire professional life. This allows me as a researcher to observe how social change occurs over time and allows me to develop frameworks that reflect changes. To demonstrate the way that research within a community can be a rewarding, challenging and evolving endeavour, I return to my home village in Ghana where the launch of an historical research project spun off into two directions of impact—one positive and one negative—and caused me to reflect on the research relationship I had developed and nurtured in my home community.

Over a period of 40 years, social research and its documentation has become a standard part of community development undertaken in my Ghanaian home village of Botoku. Research has given my village a voice and powerful tools with which to make change. But uncovering truths and questioning the status quo can be a dangerous thing and a source of conflict as well as a means for making peace. Social research, like human beings and human relationships, is often complex and unpredictable. This was made very clear to me in Botoku during a visit home in 2012 when I launched the result of a research project—a short history of Botoku from migration and settlement through to present-day social and cultural developments, commissioned by the chiefs and elders and written in collaboration with my friend and mentor, 'Colonel' Asamoah.

The book had been 10 years in the making and was launched with much laughter and fanfare. The formal launch was performed by the Minister of Tourism, a senior

© Springer Nature Switzerland AG 2019

K. Tsey, *Working on Wicked Problems*,

https://doi.org/10.1007/978-3-030-22325-0_9

member of the ruling government at the time, who comes from Botoku. The place was full of people: invited politicians and other dignitaries, school children, the *Asafos* or youth groups, church groups, music groups and the chiefs and elders in their brightly coloured clothes and paraphernalia. There were speeches, followed by music and dancing. The school cultural group performed a moving poetry recital in honour of Colonel and me for our dedication in writing a history of their beloved village. The book was priced at 10 GH cedi (US$5) a copy, and all proceeds were to go to the Botoku Education Trust. The Minister, however, did not believe that the invited dignitaries and people with financial means should buy this valuable book for 10 cedi. She considered that it would be an insult to Botoku and to the authors. So, leading by example, she paid 50 cedi ($25) for her signed copy. Then, with humour, she turned to key people in the crowd and, like an auctioneer, called for them to follow her lead and purchase their own copies. The price began at 50 cedi and, like a reverse auction, decreased to 45 and then to 40, until it came down to the basic 10 cedi. Over 350 people attended the event, and 84 copies of the history book were sold, mostly to people who paid more than the 10 cedi price as a way of contributing to the fundraising. For the next few weeks, it was gratifying to see all sorts of people, even those who could not read or write, buying the book, or sitting in small groups reading and discussing the stories and the colourful photos.

The launch and the book itself, however, were also the catalyst for two major new developments in the history of Botoku: one was the resolution of a long-running dispute about the village burial ground; the other was the start of an emotion-charged dispute between clan groups over chieftaincy in Botoku. The Botoku history book was a source of much pride and interest in the community. For this reason, I thought that when the chiefs requested a meeting with the authors several days after the book launch, they wanted to thank us. This was not quite what they had in mind! Instead they took advantage of the positive atmosphere created by the book launch to seek our help to mediate a dispute. The dispute was over burial grounds and the disposal of dead bodies, and it was tearing the community apart. Colonel and I agreed to help on the condition that everyone committed to respecting confidentiality until the case was finally settled. As I had researched and documented Botoku community development initiatives on and off for 30 years by this point, people had become familiar with my ways of working. I explained that, once more, I would carefully collect information about the steps taken towards resolving this problem but asked that everyone at the meeting help in some way so we would all learn from the process.

In Botoku, all serious business must be dealt with at dawn when, it is believed, the mind is freshest. The serious business we were about to attend to was fast escalating into a crisis. The village burial ground was full. A High Court injunction was in place preventing further burials on adjoining land. Families of terminally ill people in the village were worried. All goodwill on the part of the cemetery landowners had been exhausted. The chiefs and elders from the village had asked Colonel and me to help them break this stalemate and resolve the conflict. The meeting took place at Colonel's house. By 5 am, a large group from the village was sitting on the open veranda. There were seven male and five female chiefs, the elected district assembly representative, church leaders and the *yokufia*, or youth leader, who was responsible for digging graves and cemetery oversight.

It is customary in Botoku that land for public use is given free of charge. The village burial site had been donated to the village by one clan group 70 years earlier. The cemetery landowners claimed the community had now exhausted its original allocation and was encroaching on the land beyond it. They had applied to the High Court for an injunction to restrict further burials at the site, and this decision was creating conflict in the community. More urgently, there was the problem of what to do when next someone died. I knew that Botoku was not alone; across the world, debates were beginning (and escalating) about the best way to dispose of the bodies of loved ones in dignified ways that were also environmentally friendly. We assigned roles and jobs. Information gathering was the first task. I asked those present at the meeting to speak to people they knew from other villages to gather more information about cemeteries and changes occurring in recent times. I asked the elders to consider and reflect upon the history and customs of burials in Botoku. We agreed that, given his age, Colonel would provide background support, while I would search the Internet, talk with colleagues and friends abroad and in the village and share whatever information I found. To signify the close of the early-morning meeting, Colonel went to his room and brought out a bottle of gin. As an elder, he said he could not receive the chiefs and elders in his house and see them depart with dry throats.

Before I began gathering information, I decided I needed to convince the landowners to agree to withdraw the case from court. One of the landowners, an elder, was my cousin, and so it was not difficult for me to approach him initially. He reminded me that family decisions had to be taken collectively and arranged a time for me to meet the extended family formally. At that meeting, I explained that I had been approached to help resolve the cemetery issue and I asked them to withdraw the case from court. While they agreed that litigation was not in anybody's interests, they said that the issue involved others too, and they would need to consult among their families living outside the village. They asked me to allow them another week, and they would return with an answer.

We met again about 10 days later, and their spokesperson explained that it was not their desire to go to court at all. The story they shared added another dimension to the issue—a personal one. It had been more than 10 years since they had first informed the chiefs and elders that the original allocation of land was used up. Successive warnings to the chiefs and elders were not taken seriously. When, finally, the family gave an ultimatum to the village to stop burying on the unallocated land, people from the village, including chiefs and elders, responded with insults, name-calling and vilification. I listened carefully while they expressed their deep feelings of hurt and frustration and described the insults they had suffered. They wanted me to know now that Colonel and I had put them in an almost untenable position; their respect for us and our general standing in the community made it hard for them to say no to us. I thanked them and their family sincerely for their co-operation. They agreed to withdraw the case and, in turn, thanked me for understanding their grievances. I told them about the two conditions that Colonel and I had agreed with the chiefs: confidentiality until a final settlement was achieved and agreement that I would document the process to allow people to learn from the experience to guide the future.

Colonel and I met again with the chiefs and elders soon after. We told them the landowners had agreed to withdraw from the High Court case. I then returned to my suggestion that we step back and reflect on how Botoku had disposed of their dead in the past, consider how they were doing it now and determine whether we could learn from changes happening in similar villages or in other parts of the world. Could we find a new direction for Botoku? Talk and opinions flowed enthusiastically from the group. Everybody was keen to put across their views and share their findings, and I carefully documented them all.

Talk began with a discussion of Botoku's traditional burial practices. In the present day, concrete headstones are used, but, in the past, this was not so. When a person died, the clan group and community stayed awake overnight with the body, while information was sent to relatives and friends in the nearby villages. Preparations were made for burial to occur. The overnight watch was to protect against hyaenas trying to steal the corpse for a feast. For the burial, the body was wrapped in the dead person's favourite clothing and placed in a shallow grave. Each clan group had its own burial grounds. There were no memorials or tombstones. The only indication of a grave site was a couple of clay pots and plates in which food and water were left to sustain the dead person during the journey to the spirit world. For the Botoku people, it was sad to lose a loved one, but the dead were not considered separate from the living. Death was simply a passage that allowed humans to enter the world of the ancestors who, to this day, are ever-present in Ghanaian death rituals and practices.

All customs had changed with the arrival of Christianity. Community cemeteries where the dead were buried in timber coffins became a permanent feature in southern Ghana. Memorials were erected 1 year after the death. At first, memorials were simple wooden crosses with a concrete foundation to protect the wood from termites. Over time though, gravestones became expensive features. Nobody knew why but it became the practice to line graves with cement blocks, presumably to prevent the walls caving in. The gravestones themselves were now made of cement, and the marble headstones were becoming ever bigger. Some graves were lined with expensive marble tiles. Burials had become a contest of status as families competed to see who could build the most imposing tombstones for their loved ones. Increasingly, people were choosing aluminium caskets rather than wooden coffins because they were seen to have higher status. The rising cost of funerals was pushing many families into debt. Families who could not afford to look after their children at school or send the sick to hospital were willing to pour money into funerals. Bodies were being kept in mortuaries for months and even years so families could prepare for funerals.

This modernisation of burial practices had happened in many parts of Ghana. People in many villages were now questioning how and why their practices had changed so dramatically. Some villages and towns were now considering simple Islamic burials and funerals. Other communities had banned cement tombstones in the hope that, as in the days before Christianity, burial grounds might eventually be reused for other purposes. Other communities were planting trees for timber on burial grounds instead of gravestones, while others still were planting cassava to be processed into ethanol for clean energy. When the sharing and discussions ended, the group was agreed on one thing: if Botoku continued the way it was going, there would be no land left for their children and their children's children.

It was my turn to share what I had learned about cemetery practices and trends in the world beyond Ghana. I said that in 1850 the world's population was estimated at 1.2 billion. Within 100 years, in 1950, it had more than doubled to 2.5 billion, and by 2050, it was expected to jump nearly four times that to nine billion people. The two main forms of body disposal were burial and cremation. Population growth and shortage of land often caused people to move from burial to cremation. While the transition could be hard, necessity forced people to change. I spoke about the environmental limitations of burial and cremation: burial locked up land that could be used for other purposes and contaminated the soil through the use of embalming chemicals; cremation required smaller amounts of land but used a lot of energy and emitted carbon dioxide which contributed to atmospheric pollution.

I introduced two ideas related to disposal of bodies that had appeared in the recent past as potential ways of solving the problem. Green burials were, in many ways, a return to the way Botoku buried people before Christianity. Green burials used only biodegradable materials so that burial grounds could be reused for other purposes, including growing food crops. The second option, alkaline hydrolysis, involved placing the body in a solution of lye and water where, within a short time, it simply dissolved into liquid, including most of the bones. Remaining bones were crushed into ash and, together with the liquid, could be used as fertiliser. I said that it would take time for people to accept such new ideas but that necessity would eventually drive us to change. Long discussions about the similarities and differences between Ghana and other places followed. For example, in India cremation is the norm, but among the Botoku and central Ewe-speaking people, cremation was traditionally reserved for witches.

Following on from the discussions, things moved quickly. The court case was withdrawn, and I was given 4 weeks to report the final settlement back to the court. After the case was formally withdrawn from the court, Colonel and I succeeded in bringing the two parties together to arbitrate a settlement. As usual, we met in the early morning on Colonel's veranda. The atmosphere was very tense as the contesting parties faced each other to discuss the issue that had sharply divided the village. Formal greetings were exchanged, and I opened the meeting with a summary of our involvement in the case. I went over how the chiefs and elders had approached us, the two conditions upon which we agreed to be involved, explained my approaches to the landowners and noted our gratefulness for the respect they showed us by agreeing to withdraw the case. Next, I spoke about the work we had done to remember and reflect on Botoku's changing cultural practices. I went over the lessons to be learned, not only from our history but from other communities in Ghana and across the world. Botoku needed to be willing to adapt.

The two parties took turns expressing their perspectives. The chiefs and elders reiterated some of the key points made, while the landowners expressed frustration that a lack of respect and inaction on the part of the chiefs were largely to blame for the dispute. Then, as Botoku custom requires, we had to approach *abrewa* (a mystical old woman renowned for her wisdom) for her advice. A representative from each of the two parties, together with Colonel and me, consulted with *abrewa* in a private location. Our consultation lasted about 45 min, and we reconvened the full meeting so I could announce the key outcomes of *abrewa*'s deliberations. By custom, anything said while consulting with *abrewa* must never be divulged directly.

Firstly, *abrewa* wanted Botoku to be grateful to the landowners for their generosity in allowing the village to use their land free of charge for over 70 years. She wanted to point out to the whole of Botoku that *ewu ke to le amengo ya woduo*. Translated literally, the phrase means that a person must dance the style of dance which is fashionable at that stage in their life. The implication was that, as the world changes, so too do people, culture and practices. *Abrewa* too was unhappy with the direction in which Botoku people had gone with their cemeteries. She reminded us that even the land on which we were gathered that day had once been the burial ground for the Botoku Lobo clan group. She asked the chiefs and elders to show leadership by convincing people to rethink their burial practices. Botoku needed to think about its children's children. As our ancestors did before, people should bury their loved ones in simple ways, so future generations could reuse the land. Banning aluminium caskets and concrete gravestones would be a first step in that direction.

Abrewa said that for 12 months from the date of settlement, the landowners should continue to allow the village to bury in empty spaces within but not outside the boundaries of the original cemetery. In the meantime, the chiefs and elders should negotiate with the current landowners or others to secure land for a new cemetery. *Abrewa* wanted the entire village to know that any new plots acquired for a cemetery would necessarily require some amount of payment per burial. While every effort would be made to ensure that this did not become a burden to families, it was important to prepare the community beforehand. *Abrewa* wanted to remind everybody that opportunity often comes unexpectedly from adversity. Botoku, despite its rural isolation, had always been at the forefront of innovation and change in the district. With a pioneering role in adopting cocoa farming in the 1920s and strong achievements in education, the people had been the envy of other villages. *Abrewa* wanted everybody to take away reassurance and confidence in the Botoku people's determination and capacity to overcome conflicts and divisions. She was convinced that whatever steps the community took to resolve the cemetery dispute would be the beginning of a bigger change that would have implications for Ghana and beyond. The people should be proud of themselves for achieving peaceful resolution of their dispute. Having shared *abrewa*'s wisdom, it was my turn to provide the bottle of gin that signified the close of the meeting.

The chiefs and elders now had responsibility for working with landowners and the broader community to put *abrewa*'s directives into practice. I took photos of the typical gravestones before settlement of the dispute, so I could compare them with subsequent graves and memorials over time. At the time of writing this book, the community continues to bury the dead in the same cemetery with the consent of the landowners but for a fee of 20 cedi ($10) per burial with an additional 50 cedi charged to those people who continue to erect concrete gravestones. The extra charge is intended as a deterrent. Some landowners I spoke to were unhappy about the use of concrete tombstones by families willing to afford the extra levy but acknowledged that it was better to work with people, so they realised the need for change themselves, rather than imposing change from outside. The plan was for the Botoku Youth Association to use community versions of the story to engage the relevant groups as part of the ongoing dialogue towards the search for more sustainable funeral practices.

We had managed to capitalise on the positive atmosphere engendered by the book launch to successfully bring the parties together to make peace, but, as is often the case with research projects, there was a flip side. As community versions of the cemetery story were being prepared, a national Ghanaian newspaper carried a news headline: 'Tension in Botoku over planned enstoolment of Paramount Chief'. The same historical research that had led to the positive resolution of the cemetery dispute had facilitated, if not created, an entirely new dispute. The historical research had stirred up new disputes about which of the seven Botoku clan chiefs should be the legitimate paramount or head chief (i.e. first among equals). The matter looked like it would end up in the courts. It felt like déjà vu. The newspaper story explained how a planned coronation of a Paramount Chief for Botoku was generating tension as two factions laid claim to the title. Although the installation went ahead, its legality was (and is currently) disputed in court.

The dispute itself arose partly out of the commissioned history that the Colonel and I wrote for the village. In that book we documented how the role of paramount or head chief shifted from one clan group to another over 100 years earlier. While many people had always known the circumstances under which the paramountcy shifted from one group to the other, nobody ever questioned it. The book had changed that; as one of the parties to the dispute told me, 'Nobody cared about this story until your book put it in black and white. So the Kledzasi people [the group trying to reclaim the role] are now using it to support their claim'. The point is that whatever the outcome of the dispute, the conflict is a good example of research having an unintended impact. My own view on the matter, which I have started expressing gradually to people affected, is that we should view the dispute as an opportunity for Botoku to lead the way to democratise and reform the institution of chieftaincy in Ghan, for example, to allow men and women to have equal claims, to open the institution to all groups and not only certain families, to limit the duration of the chieftaincy to 5–10 years rather than for life and to do away with some of the obsolete and anachronistic aspects of chieftaincy rituals. The challenge for me, personally, is that I strongly believe the institution needs reforming, but I am also concerned that we do not simply replace it with western-style elections where only those with money and influence can successfully bid for elected office. It is my hope that Botoku will not only continue to work towards more sustainable burial and funeral practices but will also view the chieftaincy dispute as an opportunity for positive change.

Bibliography

Asamoah, F. M. K., & Tsey, K. (2012). *Botoku/Dzali: History, culture and governance. A learning resource for teachers, parents and students interested in African knowledge traditions.* Kwabenya: University Child and Youth Development Centre.

Tsey, K. (2011). *Re-thinking development in Africa: An oral history approach from Botoku, Rural Ghana.* Cameroon: Langaa Research & Publishing Common Initiative Group.

Tsey, K. (2018). The search for sustainable disposal of dead bodies: The case of Botoku, Rural Ghana. *OIDA International Journal of Sustainable Development, 11*(5), 23–30.

Planning for and Tracking Research Impact: Australian Research Council Framework

10

Abstract

Researchers worldwide are increasingly required to report the societal impact of their research as part of national research productivity assessments. Researchers in Aboriginal and Torres Strait Islander communities have a particularly high level of expertise in impact, which has grown out of Indigenous people's determination to take greater control and ownership of research not only to achieve benefits for the communities where the research is done but also to share the lessons with others. As a researcher, the way to prove one's worth in the research community is to demonstrate research impact. Research impact studies and the methods used to measure and report research impact are still in development. They will change and evolve. What is unlikely to change is the importance of impact reporting. This chapter examines the challenges involved in developing an impact case study for Family Wellbeing Empowerment research in the context of an Australian Research Council research impact assessment exercise. It describes the way researchers need to imagine from the outset the different types of impact their research is likely to have over the short, medium and longer terms, to enable them to plan for and record these data progressively for impact measurement and reporting, whatever form these may take.

Research impact, although we did not know it by that particular name 30 years ago, was always an overriding consideration for myself and my colleagues working in Australian Indigenous communities. Our research is not carried out for the sake of curiosity; rather, it is always based upon and built out of a wish to make a difference to people's health and wellbeing. Research impact is very difficult to demonstrate. For research impact to occur, you must show that your research outputs have influenced others to bring about changes in policy, practice or behaviour which have, in turn, resulted in some benefit to the wider society. Researchers must gather data from the point of view of users beyond academia as evidence of impact.

© Springer Nature Switzerland AG 2019
K. Tsey, *Working on Wicked Problems*,
https://doi.org/10.1007/978-3-030-22325-0_10

Planning for and gathering data that will feed into impact assessment is best done before, during and long after a research study rather than as an afterthought.

Determining whether a particular piece of research has had a beneficial impact on society is methodologically difficult, especially when researchers are being asked to undertake this exercise retrospectively. Retrospective impact assessment is complicated and may not be as reliable as one may hope if the original research project did not record the baseline data needed to consider impact. Key challenges include the time lag between conducting research and using the resultant knowledge; the difficulty in assessing and attributing the relative contribution of the many factors that combine to generate change (particularly relevant in multi-faceted social research); and the substantial cost of tracking and assessing societal impact. These challenges notwithstanding the issue of research impact have arrived, and government policy, both in Australia and internationally, is focusing the attention of researchers and their institutions more explicitly on the impact agenda.

The Australian Research Council (ARC) now requires researchers to demonstrate the impact of their research using a case study approach. The goal of the ARC impact assessment criteria is to facilitate institutional change in ways that support researchers to be more responsive to the needs of research users outside academia. The first step for researchers using the ARC criteria is to provide a clear narrative statement about their research impact, including the beneficiaries of the impact and its scope and reach. This is followed by a description of the underpinning research and the processes through which the research was used to influence decisions and practices resulting in the impact claim. To inform its approach, ARC initially called for researchers to take part in a pilot round of reporting. My team and I were interested in exploring the impact and contribution of our Family Wellbeing (FWB) research engagement in the wider community, and so we decided to put together an impact case study to contribute.

Impact has long been the starting point of research projects related to FWB. Our work has taken place in communities that had rightly expressed scepticism about research, having been 'researched to death' for many years by people and organisations that were misguided and underfunded at best, and, at worst, self-serving. Much research had occurred in Indigenous communities, but little change had taken place. I began working in these communities at a time when people were beginning to stand up and say a very clear 'no' to research if it appeared to be self-serving or irrelevant. Researchers had to be able to explain, demonstrate and prove the way that their intended research outcomes would lead to change. Knowing that I had articulated research impact achievements and goals from the start of FWB research, I surmised that producing a case study would be entirely possible. While I was correct in assuming this, some aspects of producing the case study seemed, from very early in the exercise, frighteningly difficult. The data we had collected and the parameters of our research did not fit neatly within the ARC reporting criteria. From the outset, I was concerned that we would not be able to describe FWB research impact properly and completely within the constraints of the ARC framework.

In developing the impact case study, we discovered quickly that there were two parameters in the ARC criteria that might restrict us from presenting a true and full account of the impact of FWB research. These related to timeframes and institutional affiliations. The reported research impact must have occurred between 1 January 2011 and 31 December 2016 (6 years), while the reference period for the underpinning research was 1 January 2002 to 31 December 2016 (15 years). The reported impact must also have occurred within the researcher's current institutional employment or affiliation. For our team, which collaborated widely, this was difficult. From the outset, it was clear that the requirement for reporting only research impact occurring at the researchers' current university posed serious challenges for the FWB research and translation activities. These activities had been ongoing for nearly 20 years, during which time the key researchers had changed institutions several times. We made a deliberate decision not to be constrained by this particular aspect of the ARC assessment criteria in the pilot exercise. Rather, we decided that we should use the pilot exercise as an opportunity to draw attention to the potential risks that the ARC criteria presented in constraining the capacity of researchers to demonstrate the true impact of research.

For research to have impact in wider society, the research outputs such as evidence must have been used to influence policy or practice. Further, such influence must result in social, health, economic or cultural benefit for research users outside academia. For intervention research, such as FWB, the process of demonstrating research impact became even more complex because of the need to distinguish between the impact of the program on a participant's health and wellbeing and the extent to which evidence of such health and wellbeing impact influenced FWB uptake and associated benefits in new settings. For the purposes of this chapter, the term *program impact* is used to refer to the demonstrable health and wellbeing benefits arising for individuals and communities participating in the FWB program. *Research impact*, on the other hand, refers to the process by which a particular piece of FWB evaluative research (demonstrating health and wellbeing benefits) influenced user uptake in new settings with consequential health and wellbeing benefits for the later participants and their communities.

In the early stages of this process, we contemplated contracting an independent evaluator to conduct interviews and/or focus group discussions with the communities and organisations believed to have been influenced by our research related to the FWB program. An independent assessment would minimise any perceived biases associated with the impact claims. We considered another approach too. We could articulate what we believed to be the FWB research impact and then subject the claims to an independent process of contribution tracing, a concept developed by Befani and Stedman-Bryce. Contribution tracing offers a potential method to address the challenge of identifying causality when assessing research impact, particularly for researchers in the social sciences. The method provides guidance on how to measure evidence increases/decreases and provides a mathematical measure for determining a confidence level for impact claims, whether quantitative or qualitative. Such approaches were soon discounted since we did not have dedicated resources or time to employ an independent assessor to collect and process new data for the pilot exercise. Hence, we decided that the research team, in collaboration with the relevant industry partners previously involved in FWB evaluations, would conduct the impact assessment based on existing project data with a commitment to making the process as transparent as possible. To this end, we enlisted the assistance of a senior research policy analyst and manager who was not familiar with the FWB research and provided the perspective of an outsider (i.e. a critical friend). We had been noting the impact of FWB research in one form or another since the project began and were confident we could begin with these data.

There were many arms of FWB throughout the country and overseas, and the program had spread and evolved over many years. Much of the uptake could be traced back to the FWB research evaluation project carried out in Alice Springs in 1998–1999 and to the enquiries and interest generated through the scholarly outputs from the research evaluation. We were able to demonstrate the reach and growth of FWB through a broader empowerment research program, involving several Indigenous organisations. We used the enthusiasm and demand for FWB generated by the Alice Springs evaluation (described in Chap. 6) to create the 10-year empowerment research program in 2002 to assess the role and contribution of empowerment in enabling Indigenous people to take greater control and responsibility for their health. We focused on initiatives that Indigenous people themselves labelled as empowerment or self-determination projects, including FWB, community-controlled organisations and men's, women's and youth groups. FWB was tailored to address different issues in different locations: youth suicide prevention, men's and women's support group issues, family violence, mental health, youth sexual health, child protection, the resilience of school students, leadership, workforce development, organisational change in community-controlled services and university-level soft skills courses. The Aboriginal-developed program had spread internationally to 60 known sites and been delivered in workshops to more than 3500 participants since its development in 1992. The empowerment research program motivated many researchers to embark on long-term research and translation activities in support of FWB program uptake and evaluation in new settings and dozens of published FWB impact evaluation papers; the empowerment research program produced papers that theorised about the meaning of empowerment for Indigenous Australians, described university-community research partnerships and models of research capacity strengthening and discussed the transferability and uptake of empowerment programs across Australia. The papers also included descriptions of tools produced to measure psychosocial empowerment and wellbeing.

For the ARC impact assessment case study, we looked at FWB program delivery in sites like Yarrabah, where the programs and research had been ongoing for up to 20 years, and in other sites where FWB was delivered in a one-off capacity. We carefully reviewed a range of available resources that reflected user perspectives and other independent assessments of the value of FWB research. These included media releases and personal and professional reflections by FWB participants and service providers using the program. We also looked at annual reports, research reports, media appearances, community FWB promotional videos and independent reviews of Indigenous intervention research citing FWB publications. We conducted a co-author network analysis based on 48 published FWB evaluations produced by our research team to determine the extent of Indigenous and industry participation in the research. Essentially, we researched our research.

In the case of Yarrabah, FWB had empowered the community in a way that helped to build a foundational social health workforce and translate their vision for a community-controlled health service into reality. From the time FWB first came to Yarrabah in 2001, employee numbers at the new health service went from 2 to more than 70 by 2016–88% of whom were local Indigenous people. While these developments could not be seen as a direct outcome of the FWB research, community members considered FWB as a catalyst for change. In Yarrabah we were able to document population-level or whole-of-community benefits arising from the ongoing research collaboration. These included the development of the community's local social health workforce largely out of people who, until that time, had been on unemployment benefits. The FWB intervention had empowered people at a personal level to make changes like pursuing employment and further education. The growth in jobs and people's employment capabilities was so significant that it had an impact on the community itself. Changes in the community included a notable reduction in suicide rates, and this has been maintained since the early 2000s. This was in addition to the usual improved social and emotional wellbeing protective factors that were documented among FWB participants themselves.

The impact findings we were able to demonstrate in Yarrabah, however, contrasted with a number of other communities where evaluative research with FWB had taken place without the long-term two-step Participatory Action Research that had occurred in Yarrabah. In some communities FWB was applied more simply—to empower individuals to meet their own personal needs more effectively. It was not used as a catalyst to generate ideas or actions for wider change. In these settings, it was not possible to demonstrate impact beyond the usual individual social and emotional wellbeing benefits. By way of example, the Central Coast Primary Care service (CCPC) in Gosford, New South Wales, adopted FWB as a personal empowerment model only. Between 2012 and 2019, the service team delivered 10-week FWB programs to over 300 young men (98% were Indigenous). The evaluation reported statistically significant improvements in psychosocial wellbeing among the FWB participants before and after participation. Participants' feedback was also positive, for example, 'Since I started the program I have learnt and achieved a lot of skills to help change my life for the better and it has been a great experience' and 'The family wellbeing program helped me to be good at school and a heaps better person in general'. Delivery of the FWB program within the community was extensive, but it had not driven further research or built research capacity at a community level. From a comparison of the two impact case studies in Yarrabah and Gosford, it was clear that broader population-level impact required a long-term, two-step approach, which was based on rolling evaluation, review and revision.

A social network analysis was conducted to capture the relational nature of FWB research. This analysis demonstrated that the university-based researchers were affiliated with 12 different universities and that FWB programs had been conducted with 12 industry partners in a variety of contexts and locations in 4 countries: Australia (88%), PNG (8%), China (2%) and Timor-Leste (2%). The analysis revealed the longevity of the research team as a critical factor in facilitating FWB uptake. Although the researchers were affiliated with different organisations and universities, their commitment to the research intervention was consistent and long-standing. Four key authors were identified: Tsey (44 papers since 2000), Whiteside (24 papers since 2003), McCalman (17 papers since 2005) and Cadet-James (12 papers since 2004). These authors have co-authored papers for more than 10 years and have collaborated with many industry and university authors, with 62 individual authors named across the total publications. For most of these collaborations, potential users had heard of or read one FWB paper and then enquired directly of the author. The enquiries made after reading an FWB research paper, and the responsiveness of FWB researchers in supporting program uptake and evaluation in new settings, contributed to the research impact claims.

Managers at the CCPC, discussed earlier, explained in an FWB newsletter story how they had encountered the FWB empowerment program when conducting a literature search in 2012. Managers had been searching for culturally appropriate social and emotional wellbeing programs targeting Indigenous youth at risk of dropping out of school or entering the juvenile justice system. After reading the evaluation of the 1998–1999 Alice Springs FWB project, they made contact with me and my team. The body of evidence, accumulated over a 10-year period of FWB evaluative research, which I shared with the CCPC health service, convinced them to invite the FWB research team to help implement and evaluate the program across their service catchment area. The FWB CCPC case example revealed that it can take many years—13 in this case—for research to be taken up in a new setting and an additional 1 or 2 years for short-term pre-intervention and post-intervention impacts to be observed.

Both the Yarrabah and CCPC examples contained evidence demonstrating wider research impact of the FWB program, but they simply did not meet the ARC pilot criteria in their current form. In the CCPC case, the 1998–1999 evaluative research, conducted at the time I was with Menzies School of Health Research in Alice Springs, influenced uptake in 2012. This disqualified the case study outright because it fell outside the ARC's 15-year reference period, and I was no longer at Menzies. Although the Yarrabah uptake was also influenced by the 1998–1999 study, the research partnership with that community has been longer and has been sustained since 2001. This provided some flexibility to present FWB research activities in that community since 2002 as associated or underpinning research. Nevertheless, the final case study focused mainly on improved wellbeing among program participants, not on population-level suicide prevention impacts that occurred prior to the transfer of the FWB program of research from The University of Queensland to James Cook University. The constraints of institutional affiliation and specified assessment timeframes thus significantly diminished reporting of what we believed to be the true impact of the FWB research and translation activities. Not surprisingly, the FWB research impact case we submitted under the ARC's 2018 assessment round received 'high' for 'approach' to impact but 'medium' for 'impact' itself on a rating scale of high medium and low.

We could show that participation in the FWB empowerment program had consistently led to improvements in the health and social wellbeing of Indigenous Australians. The Productivity Commission, in its 2016 Closing the Gap report on Indigenous disadvantage to Parliament, cited FWB, based on our research, as a cultural healing program and a 'thing that works' to promote community functioning. Systematic literature reviews commissioned by Beyond Blue and the Sax Institute identified FWB as one of only five promising Indigenous Australian social and emotional wellbeing programs and as a cultural approach to trauma-specific care. The impacts for participants were numerous and included increased capacity to exert greater control over health and wellbeing, a heightened sense of identity, respect for self and others, enhanced parenting, newfound capacity to deal with substance abuse and violence, improved life skills, connectedness and belonging, confidence to recognise and intervene in potential suicide and a significant reduction in distress. Participants' improvements influenced other individuals and, over time, systems, highlighting the ecological dimensions of empowerment. These skills, fostered in individuals but translating also to families and community groups, constituted powerful protective factors for health and wellbeing.

Our primary concern regarding FWB research was, and still is, to find compelling qualitative and quantitative ways in which to demonstrate the costs versus benefits of implementing the FWB program on a wider scale. We started the evaluation process with Indigenous notions of story-telling (described in Chap. 6) to develop deep understandings of the program theory, impact and context, which we used to develop scales to quantify pre- and post-intervention wellbeing outcomes and cost analysis. Based on FWB and other related research experiences, my team and I collaborated with the Lowitja Institute to develop a Research for Impact Tool designed to assist researchers to plan for and assess the impact of their research from the beginning rather than at the end of their projects. The premise of the tool is that the value of research is to create evidence and/or products to help decision makers, whether they be governments, businesses, service providers or households, to make smarter decisions that can have knock-on effects in improving the human condition. Figure 10.1 is an overview of the Research for Impact Tool. It illustrates the steps researchers can take to plan for and track impact by first defining their research priorities, identifying potential research users and determining their evidence needs. The next step is considering whether existing knowledge is adequate to inform users' decisions or if additional evidence is required. This initial planning is followed by steps associated with ensuring the research type and design are fit for purpose; assessing the wellbeing, economic, social and cultural benefits versus costs; translating the knowledge produced to influence decisions and actions beyond the project; and, finally, assessing the overall costs and benefits of the research and translation activities, both intended and unintended. Embedded at each step is the need for research leadership and participation, research capacity enhancement, equity (e.g. fairness, justness), diversity (e.g. gender, early career research) and a commitment to learning by doing.

A key premise of our tool is that researchers need to start by finding out the information needs of users and then use existing or new research to help meet these information needs in a timely fashion. Many researchers look for gaps in the

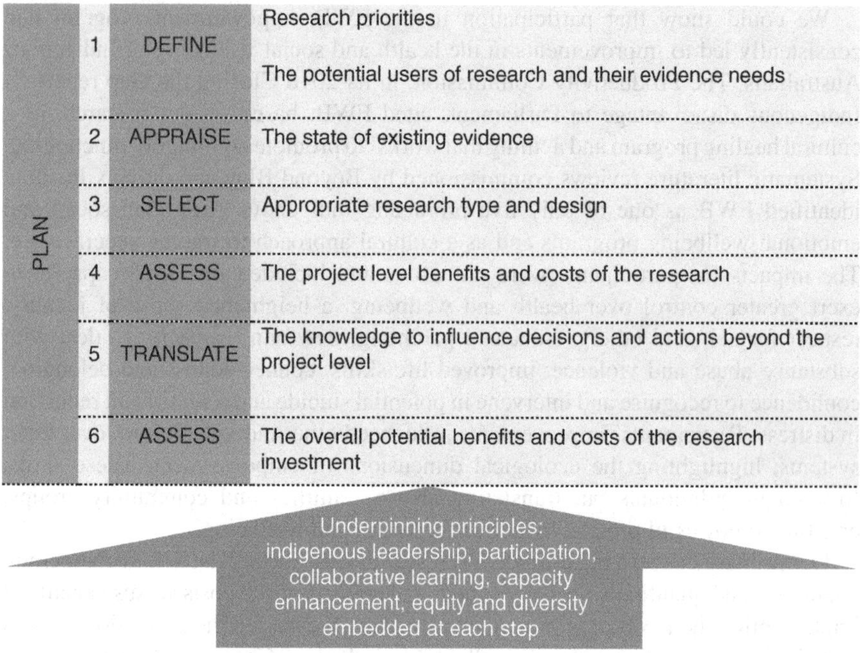

	1	DEFINE	Research priorities The potential users of research and their evidence needs
PLAN	2	APPRAISE	The state of existing evidence
	3	SELECT	Appropriate research type and design
	4	ASSESS	The project level benefits and costs of the research
	5	TRANSLATE	The knowledge to influence decisions and actions beyond the project level
	6	ASSESS	The overall potential benefits and costs of the research investment

Underpinning principles: indigenous leadership, participation, collaborative learning, capacity enhancement, equity and diversity embedded at each step

Fig. 10.1 Research for Impact Tool

research evidence base to fill, rather than considering the needs of their research communities as the highest priority. An unmet need is more than a gap in the evidence; identifying an unmet need is usually the first step in creating meaningful research. In other words, *information needs* rather than *information gaps* should be the drivers of social research. In seeking to develop and measure research with impact, researchers need to imagine the impact their research is likely to have, in all its various forms (health and wellbeing, economic, social, cultural), over the short, medium and longer terms, and put templates in place to record data pre-emptively rather than retrospectively. Researchers must also maintain a flexible approach to ensure optimal methods are developed over time, enabling rather than constraining the capacity of researchers to demonstrate the true impact of their research, both intended and unintended.

Bibliography

Australian Research Council. (2017a). Engagement and impact assessment pilot 2017. Australian Research Council. Retrieved December 18, 2018, from http://www.arc.gov.au/sites/default/files/filedepot/Public/EI/Engagement_and_Impact_Assessment_Pilot_2017_Report.pdf. Accessed 18 December 2018.

Australian Research Council. (2017b). EI 2018 Submission guidelines. Australian Research Council. Retrieved December 18, 2018, from http://www.arc.gov.au/sites/default/files/filedepot/Public/EI/EI_2018_Submission_Guidelines.pdf.

Befani, B., & Stedman-Bryce, G. (2017). Process tracing and Bayesian updating for impact evaluation. *Evaluation, 23*(1), 42–60.

Brown, C. (2010). What's in it for me? My story of becoming a facilitator of an Aboriginal Empowerment Program. *Aboriginal and Islander Health Worker Journal, 34*(5), 12.

Brown, C. (2011). You get help and you give help: My role as an Aboriginal Family Wellbeing facilitator. *Aboriginal and Islander Health Worker Journal, 35*, 24–28.

Gibson, T. (2004). Family wellbeing: My story. *Aboriginal and Islander Health Worker Journal, 28*(6), 3–5.

Haswell, M. R., Kavanagh, D., Tsey, K., Reilly, L., Cadet-James, Y., Laliberte, A., et al. (2010). Psychometric validation of the Growth and Empowerment Measure (GEM) applied with Indigenous Australians. *Australian and New Zealand Journal of Psychiatry, 44*(9), 791–799. https://doi.org/10.3109/00048674.2010.482919.

Heyeres, M., Tsey, K., Yang, Y., Yan, L., & Jiang, H. (2018). The characteristics and reporting quality of research impact case studies: A systematic review. *Evaluation and Program Planning, 73*, 10–23. https://doi.org/10.1016/j.evalprogplan.2018.11.002.

Kinchin, I., Doran, C. M., McCalman, J., Jacups, S., Tsey, K., Lines, K., et al. (2017a). Delivering an empowerment intervention to a remote Indigenous child safety workforce: Its economic cost from an agency perspective. *Evaluation and Program Planning, 64*, 85–89. https://doi.org/10.1016/j.evalprogplan.2017.05.017.

Kinchin, I., Jacups, S., Tsey, K., & Lines, K. (2015). An empowerment intervention for Indigenous communities: An outcome assessment. *BMC Psychology, 3*(29). https://doi.org/10.1186/s40359-015-0086-z.

Kinchin, I., McCalman, J., Bainbridge, R., Tsey, K., & Watkin Lui, F. (2017b). Does Indigenous health research have impact? A systematic review of reviews. *International Journal for Equity in Health, 16*(1), 52. https://doi.org/10.1186/s12939-017-0548-4.

Kitau, R., Whiteside, M., Kinchin, I., Hane-Nou, G., & Tsey, K. (2017). Transferring the Aboriginal Australian family wellbeing empowerment program from a Papua New Guinea University context to broader community settings: A feasibility study. *Pacific Journal of Medical Sciences, 17*(1), 22–37.

McCalman, J., Bainbridge, R., Brown, C., Tsey, K., & Clarke, A. (2018). The Aboriginal Australian Family Wellbeing program: A historical analysis of the conditions that enabled its spread. *Frontiers in Public Health, 6*, 26. https://doi.org/10.3389/fpubh.2018.00026.

McCalman, J., Tsey, K., Reilly, L., Connolly, B., Fagan, R., Earles, W., et al. (2010). Taking control of health: Gurriny's story of organisational change. *Third Sector Review, 16*, 29–47.

McCalman, J. R. (2013). The transfer and implementation of an Aboriginal Australian wellbeing program: A grounded theory study. *Implementation Science, 8*, 1–9. https://doi.org/10.1186/1748-5908-8-129.

McEwan, A. B., Tsey, K., McCalman, J., & Travers, H. J. (2010). Empowerment and change management in Aboriginal organisations: A case study. *Australian Health Review, 34*(3), 360–367. https://doi.org/10.1071/AH08696.

Onnis, L., Klieve, H., & Tsey, K. (2018). The evidence needed to demonstrate impact: A synthesis of the evidence from a phased social and emotional wellbeing intervention. *Evaluation and Program Planning, 70*, 35–43. https://doi.org/10.1016/j.evalprogplan.2018.05.003.

Prince, J., Jeffrey, N., Baird, L., Kingsburra, S., & Tipiloura, B. (2018). Stories from community: How suicide rates fell in two Indigenous communities. Canberra: Aboriginal & Torres Strait Islander Healing Foundation.

Tsey, K. (2015). A brighter future for life in the tropics: Translating big picture academic vision into practical research. *Journal of Tropical Psychology, 5*, 1–4. https://doi.org/10.1017/jtp.2015.7.

Tsey, K., & Every, A. (2000). Evaluating Aboriginal empowerment programs: The case of Family WellBeing. *Australian and New Zealand Journal of Public Health, 24*(5), 509–514.

Tsey, K., Lawson, K., Kinchin, I., Bainbridge, R., McCalman, J., Watkin, F., Cadet-James, Y., & Rossetto, A. (2016). Evaluating research impact: The development of a 'RESEARCH for IMPACT' TOOL. *Frontiers in Public Health, 4*, 160. https://doi.org/10.3389/fpubh.2016.00160.

Tsey, K., Lui, S. M. (Carrie), Heyeres, M., Yan, L., & Pryce, J. (2018). Developing soft skills: Exploring the feasibility of an Australian Well-being program for health managers and leaders in Timor-Leste. *SAGE Open, 8*(4), 1–13. https://doi.org/10.1177/2158244018811404.

Tsey, K., Onnis, L. A., Whiteside, M., McCalman, J., Lui, S. M. C., Klieve, H., et al. (2019). Assessing research impact, Australian Research Council criteria and the case of Family Wellbeing research. *Program Planning and Evaluation, 73*, 176–186.

Tsey, K., Whiteside, M., Daly, S., Deemal, A., Gibson, T., Cadet-James, Y., et al. (2005). Adapting the 'family wellbeing' empowerment program to the needs of remote Indigenous school children. *Australian and New Zealand Journal of Public Health, 29*(2), 112–116. https://doi.org/10.1111/j.1467-842X.2005.tb00059.x.

Tsey, K., Wilson, A., Haswell-Elkins, M., Whiteside, M., McCalman, J., Cadet-James, Y., et al. (2007). Empowerment-based research methods: A 10-year approach to enhancing Indigenous social and emotional wellbeing. *Australasian Psychiatry, 15*, S34–S38. https://doi.org/10.1080/10398560701701163.

Whiteside, M., Bould, E., Tsey, K., Venville, A., Cadet-James, Y., & Morris, M. E. (2017). Promoting twenty-first-century student competencies: A wellbeing approach. *Australian Social Work, 70*(3), 324–336. https://doi.org/10.1080/0312407X.2016.1263351.

Whiteside, M., Klieve, H., Millgate, N., Webb, B., Gabriel, Z., McPherson, L., et al. (2016). Connecting and strengthening young Aboriginal men: A family wellbeing pilot study. *Australian Social Work, 69*(2), 241–252.

Whiteside, M., MacLean, S., Callinan, S., Marshall, P., Nolan, S., & Tsey, K. (2018). Acceptability of an Aboriginal wellbeing intervention for supporters of people using methamphetamines. *Australian Social Work, 71*(3), 358–366. https://doi.org/10.1080/0312407X.2018.1473455.

Whiteside, M., Tsey, K., Cadet-James, Y., & McCalman, J. (2014). *Promoting Aboriginal health: The family wellbeing empowerment approach.* New York: Springer Science & Business Media.

Whiteside, M., Tsey, K., & Earles, W. (2011). Locating empowerment in the context of Indigenous Australia. *Australian Social Work, 64*, 113–129. https://doi.org/10.1080/03124 07X.2010.533279.

Whiteside, M., Tsey, K., McCalman, J., Cadet-James, Y., & Wilson, A. (2006). Empowerment as a framework for Indigenous workforce development and organisational change. *Australian Social Work, 59*, 422–434. https://doi.org/10.1080/03124070600985996.

Yan, L., Yinghong, Y., Lui, S. M., Whiteside, M., & Tsey, K. (2018). Teaching "soft skills" to university students in China: The feasibility of an Australian approach. *Educational Studies*, 1–17. https://doi.org/10.1080/03055698.2018.1446328.

Zuchowski, I., Miles, D., Gair, S., & Tsey, K. (2019). Social work research with industry: A systematic literature review of engagement and impact. *The British Journal of Social Work*, 1–26. https://doi.org/10.1093/bjsw/bcz015.

Conclusion: A Strengths-Based Framework for Research Engagement and Impact

11

Abstract

In reviewing the research engagement and impact literature with colleagues, I found that publications to date have focused mainly on descriptions of assessment tools, templates and frameworks as well as reported impact case studies. There has not been so much focus on the values and competencies necessary for effective and emotionally safe engagement; yet this is one of the most important aspects of the work of a social researcher seeking to make a real impact through research. Researchers are dealing with increasingly complex and sensitive problems such as the ones explored in this book. It is one thing to have a theoretical framework to guide practice but quite another thing altogether to know how to put the framework into practice. Effective practice depends on having the competencies and capabilities to engage with people, work to their and your own strengths and share your findings and experiences with people who will help to enable or facilitate wider change. This chapter brings together the lessons from the various chapters of the book to present a strengths-based engagement and impact framework to guide practice, highlight the underpinning qualities and competencies required by researchers and suggest training packages to foster such competencies.

There is a growing recognition that we live in a world that is becoming more complex, rapidly changing and uncertain, with no straightforward or easy solutions to problems. Tensions include the need, given the earth's finite resources, to live our lives in a way that does not disadvantage others in our own or future generations. Societies and individuals struggle to heal from the trauma and hurt resulting from prejudice, colonisation and discriminatory practices and to reconcile with people we have historically viewed as our oppressors. Drug and alcohol misuse and associated violence, abuse and suicide afflict our communities. There is the question of how to enjoy our relatively affluent lifestyles in the midst of social inequality and

K. Tsey, *Working on Wicked Problems*,
https://doi.org/10.1007/978-3-030-22325-0_11

the growing epidemic of obesity, chronic disease, worry, stress, anxiety and illness resulting from modern busy lives. Researchers working on these wicked problems must now engage with communities in a way that goes well beyond the traditional action research and quality improvement processes of brainstorming issues, identifying indicators against which to assess performance, devising strategies and actions, implementing actions and reflecting on the outcomes. Social researchers must foster within themselves and their research participants the human qualities that are at the core of self-realisation, such as empathy, intuition, creativity, mediation, courage, forgiveness, self-awareness and analytic skills, and the application of these qualities to manage the big and small challenges and opportunities of life.

Our discipline-specific hard skills, such as analysis, statistical expertise, computing, education, nursing, sociology, economics and project management, get us into jobs and bring us research projects. Our soft skills help us to advance and enjoy a happy and successful life. Evidence suggests that up to 75% of success in long-term work and life depends on soft skills, with only 25% dependent on technical or hard skills. This research finding is also relevant to the process of research. The types of soft skills and capacities identified in the mainstream literature are the same ones the Aboriginal Family Wellbeing (FWB) program seeks to foster among participants. As teachers and researchers, we need to better understand the nature of these soft skills and how best to foster their development in our students. Strengths-based approaches set out explicitly to work with the capacity, skills, knowledge, connections and potential in individuals and communities. Strengths-based approaches are concerned largely with two factors: the quality of the relationship between researcher and research community and the quality of input the community contributes to the process. The problems and difficulties of individuals or communities are not ignored in this approach. Instead, the focus is on the people's resources and strengths, applied in a positive way, so that they can utilise these strengths to address the challenges arising from their problems. Strengths-based researchers do not ask, 'What is the problem and how can it be fixed?' Rather, they ask, 'What is working, despite the challenges, and how can we enable these effective elements to generate change and new growth?'

The role of the social researcher is to facilitate or guide the research community to work together efficiently to achieve a specific outcome without dictating the solution. A research facilitator needs sound skills in conflict resolution, active listening, reflecting, skilful questioning, linking ideas and people and ability to challenge with care. Facilitators should be able to engage participants actively, be accepting of others, show empathy, keep participants focused and make sure discussions are on target. A facilitator wears the hats of motivator, guide, questioner, bridge-builder, clairvoyant, peacemaker, taskmaster and praiser. In addition, effective facilitators must have a caring persona and be able to put their egos aside to behave merely as a servant to the group. These are all qualities that Wilkinson refers to as the 'soul' of a facilitator. The FWB foundational training helps people to identify these qualities and their own basic human needs as critical resources in generating change. It is a simple but powerful engagement tool. People reflect on the human qualities they admire in others and in themselves and correlate these with basic human physical, mental, emotional and spiritual needs. They recognise these qualities as resources available to them, and they recognise unmet human needs as barriers to the effective use of these resources.

At the time I was finishing this book, my friend Les Baird and I ran an FWB workforce development workshop for staff and managers of an Aboriginal community-controlled service. We asked everybody to identify one person in the workplace they admired. Of the 23 people at the workshop, almost a quarter of them nominated the cleaner, a young man in his late 20s. The reasons they gave included these statements: 'He is so positive'; 'His presence diffuses tension even among the professional staff'; 'He does his work with enthusiasm'; 'I heard him telling his friends that making the place clean and beautiful for staff and clients to enjoy makes him happy'; and 'His approach to life reminds me not to take myself too seriously all the time'. The cleaner had a particular mindset or approach to life that marked him out as someone whose presence and qualities were different from others. Positive psychologists call it a 'flourishing mindset'; innovation and enterprise researchers call it a 'mindset of creativity, initiative and self-reliance'. People who have this mindset view problems as opportunities for learning and growth and are able to take advantage of the opportunities that come their way. I call it an 'empowered mindset'.

There is a growing body of evidence, from fields such as neuroscience, that support the basic premise of FWB: that cultivating and using positive human qualities can promote wellbeing and teach people how to help themselves and then help others. Promoting and maintaining wellbeing is ongoing, a life-long work that needs to be monitored and measured over time. FWB empowers participants through personal transformation that involves harmonising the physical, emotional, mental and spiritual aspects of life and applying this to practical, day-to-day living. The program has been applied in various contexts and delivered to men, women, school children, adolescents, prisoners and people affected by alcohol and substance misuse. We delivered FWB in the context of workforce development and suicide prevention interventions and in international settings such as health promotion in Papua New Guinea and soft skills leadership training in Timor-Leste and China. All participants consistently report on changed mindsets and the attainment of new skills that help them to reduce stress and better handle the challenges of daily life.

Findings from FWB research correlate with research on positive mindsets, showing that people who experience and express positive emotions tend to be more resilient, resourceful and socially connected. A positive mindset affects people's behavioural and lifestyle choices. A positive mindset also arouses measurable physiological effects. When a critical mass of people has attained the skills and capabilities they need to help themselves, they will tend to help others too. Communities begin to flourish, and stronger communities have a greater capacity to deal with complex and sensitive challenges such as suicide prevention, drugs, alcohol abuse and violence. I have used insights from these engagement experiences to work as part of teams to create knowledge translation short courses and tailored follow-up support for researchers, community leaders and human services managers seeking to translate research into practice in order to enhance the impact of their work and to evaluate their practice. These courses include Introduction to Research Engagement and Impact Assessment; Building 'soft skills' for Community Engagement; and Introduction to the Family Wellbeing empowerment intervention.

Research engagement and impact are two sides of a coin. The more genuinely researchers engage, the higher their chances of achieving impact. The reverse is also true in the sense that the less meaningful the engagement, the lower the chances of demonstrating research impact. Based on the stories contained in this book, Fig. 11.1 shows a strengths-based research engagement and impact framework. Researchers must engage effectively with research partners in order to demonstrate the impact of their research, and this is at the core or the centre of the framework. 'Strengths-based facilitation' which is the role of the researcher as facilitator, supporting and guiding individuals and groups to be agents of their own change, forms a circle immediately around engagement and impact in the framework. Forming an outer

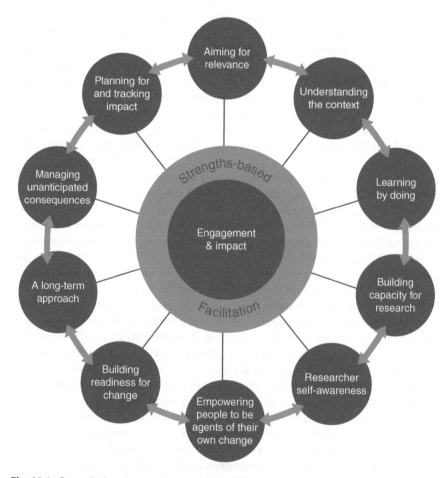

Fig. 11.1 Strengths-based research engagement and impact framework

circle around the strengths-based facilitation are the factors that enable the process of research engagement and impact, based on Chaps. 1–10:

1. Aiming for relevance
2. Understanding the context
3. Learning by doing
4. Building capacity for research
5. Building self-awareness as researcher
6. Empowering people to be agents of their own change
7. Building readiness for change
8. Taking a long-term approach
9. Managing unanticipated consequences
10. Planning for and tracking impact

The lines linking each of the ten enabling factors in the outer circle, as well as linking each factor back to the centre of the model, show the interconnectedness of the framework. Theoretical frameworks such as this are always evolving and changing based on practice. Rather than being rigidly applied, researchers and partners should adapt and tailor the framework flexibly to the needs of research settings.

Bibliography

Banerjee, P., & Puri, A. (2018). *Enhancing health and transforming lives through optimism attitude model (OAM): Panacea in 21st century*. London: The Academy of Business and Retail Management. Retrieved December 2, 2018, from https://search-proquest-com.elibrary.jcu.edu. au/docview/2089762146?accountid=16285.

Crum, A. J., Leibowitz, K. A., & Verghese, A. (2017). Making mindset matter. *British Medical Journal, 356*, j674. Retrieved December 4, 2018, from https://www.bmj.com/content/356/bmj. j674.

Finniss, D. G., Kaptchuk, T. J., Miller, F., & Benedetti, F. (2010). Placebo effects: Biological, clinical and ethical advances. *Lancet, 375*(9715), 686. Retrieved December 6, 2018, from https://www.ncbi.nlm.nih.gov/pmc/articles/PMC2832199/.

Foundation for Young Australians. (2017). The New Work Mindset. 7 new job clusters to help young people navigate the new work order. Report. Retrieved December 14, 2018, from https://www.fya.org.au/wp-content/uploads/2016/11/The-New-Work-Mindset.pdf.

Fredrickson, B. L. (2001). The role of positive emotions in positive psychology: The broaden-and-build theory of positive emotions. *American Psychologist, 56*(3), 218.

Fredrickson, B. L. (2013). Positive emotions broaden and build. *Advances in Experimental Social Psychology, 47*, 1–53. Retrieved December 14, 2018, from http://peplab.web.unc.edu/ files/2018/11/fredricskonAESP2013.pdf.

Geia, L. K., Hayes, B., & Usher, K. (2011). A strengths based approach to Australian Aboriginal childrearing practices is the answer to better outcomes in Aboriginal family and child health. *Collegian, 18*(3), 99–100.

Hammond, W. (2010). Principles of strength-based practice. *Resiliency Initiatives, 12*(2), 1–7. Retrieved December 9, 2018, from http://www.ayscbc.org/Principles%20of%20Strength-2.pdf.

Heyeres, M., Tsey, K., Yang, Y., Yan, L., & Jiang, H. (2018). The characteristics and reporting quality of research impact case studies: A systematic review. *Evaluation and Program Planning, 73*, 10–23. https://doi.org/10.1016/j.evalprogplan.2018.11.002.

Kinchin, I., McCalman, J., Bainbridge, R., Tsey, K., & Watkin Lui, F. (2017). Does Indigenous health research have impact? A systematic review of reviews. *International Journal for Equity in Health, 16*. https://doi.org/10.1186/s12939-017-0548-4.

Park, N., & Peterson, C. (2006). Moral competence and character strengths among adolescents: The development and validation of the Values in Action Inventory of Strengths for Youth. *Journal of Adolescence, 29*(6), 891–909. Retrieved December 14, 2018, from https://www.sciencedirect.com/science/article/pii/S0140197106000479.

Peters, G. B. (2017). What is so wicked about wicked problems? A conceptual analysis and research program. *Policy and Society, 36*(3), 385–396.

Prince, J., Jeffrey, N., Baird, L., Kingsburra, S., & Tipiloura, B. (2018). Stories from community: How suicide rates fell in two Indigenous communities. Canberra: Aboriginal & Torres Strait Islander Healing Foundation.

Richie, B. (2018). Challenges incarcerated women face as they return to their communities: Findings from life history interviews. In D. Hatton & A. Fisher (Eds.) Women prisoners and health justice: Perspectives, issues and advocacy for an international hidden population. (pp. 23–44). Florida: CRC Press.

Tsey, K., Lui, S. M. (Carrie), Heyeres, M., Yan, L., & Pryce, J. (2018). Developing soft skills: Exploring the feasibility of an Australian well-being program for health managers and leaders in Timor-Leste. *SAGE Open, 8*(4), 1–13. https://doi.org/10.1177/2158244018811404.

Tsey, K., Patterson, D., Whiteside, M., Baird, L., Baird, B., & Tsey, K. (2004). A microanalysis of a participatory action research process with a rural Aboriginal men's health group. *Australian Journal of Primary Health, 10*(1), 64–71. Retrieved December 12, 2018, from http://www.publish.csiro.au/py/PY04009.

Tugade, M. M., Fredrickson, B. L., & Feldman Barrett, L. (2004). Psychological resilience and positive emotional granularity: Examining the benefits of positive emotions on coping and health. *Journal of Personality, 72*(6), 1161–1190.

Wardale, D. (2013). Towards a model of effective group facilitation. *Leadership & Organization Development Journal, 34*(2), 112–129. Retrieved December 12, 2018, from https://www-emeraldinsight-com.elibrary.jcu.edu.au/doi/full/10.1108/01437731311321896.

Whiteside, M., Bould, E., Tsey, K., Venville, A., Cadet-James, Y., & Morris, M. E. (2017). Promoting twenty-first-century student competencies: A wellbeing approach. *Australian Social Work, 70*(3), 324–336. https://doi.org/10.1080/0312407X.2016.1263351.

Wilkinson, M. (2012). *The secrets of facilitation: The SMART guide to getting results with groups.* New York: John Wiley & Sons. Retrieved December 12, 2018, from https://ebookcentral.proquest.com/lib/jcu/detail.action?docID=234198.

Yan, L., Yinghong, Y., Lui, S. M., Whiteside, M., & Tsey, K. (2018). Teaching "soft skills" to university students in China: The feasibility of an Australian approach. *Educational Studies,* 1–17. https://doi.org/10.1080/03055698.2018.1446328.

Zuchowski, I., Miles, D., Gair, S., & Tsey, K. (2019). Social work research with industry: A systematic literature review of engagement and impact. *The British Journal of Social Work,* 1–26. https://doi.org/10.1093/bjsw/bcz015.

Printed in the United States
By Bookmasters